THE

breathwork

COMPANION

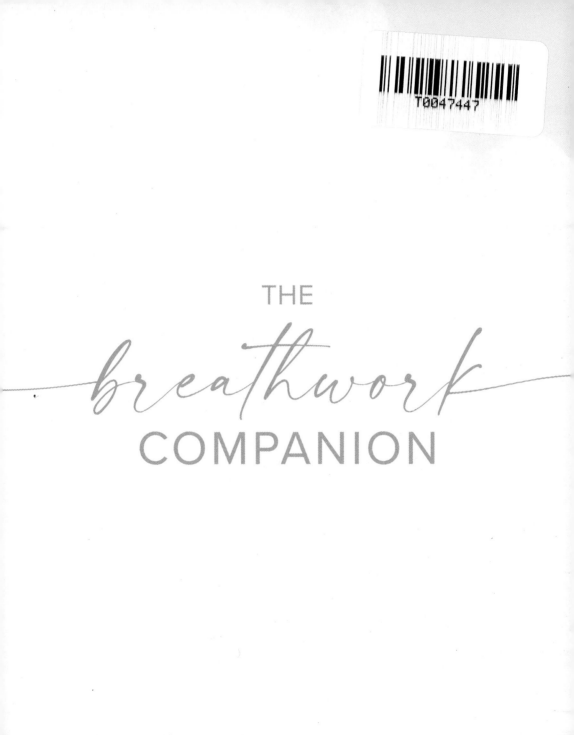

THE

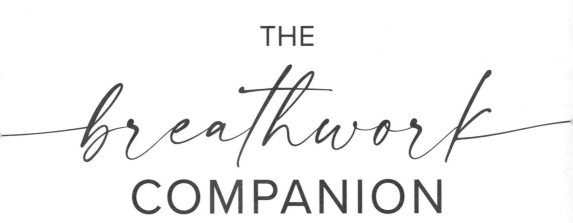

breathwork

COMPANION

Unlock the Healing
Power of Breathing

Margaret Townsend

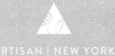

ARTISAN | NEW YORK

Contents

To be present is where you find your inner peace. Find your breath, and you are present. Stay, breathe freely, and realize a life that will carry you.

—MARGARET TOWNSEND

Introduction

This book is an invitation to breathe—better, healthier, easier, fuller, and freer.

Your breath is your body's "reset button," available to you whenever you need it. I wrote this book to share the powerful experience of the breath and the miracle of how it works, with you, in a practical and mindful way. You don't need to be a breathwork expert or a yogi to nourish your body with breath. All you need are lungs and a curiosity about how the breath affects the body and your state of awareness.

As a certified breathwork practitioner, I've been helping clients and students access the inherent healing power of the breath for more than thirty years. Breathing consciously is giving yourself nourishment—it's a gesture of self-kindness. Although you may not have given your breath acknowledgment and attention until now, it's great that you've taken the step of picking up this book. Working with the breath will make an essential difference in your life. The breath is your life force—the foundation of your physical and mental health. The way you're breathing at any given moment is influencing the way you experience life. And whatever you're experiencing affects your breath. It goes both ways.

Let's ease in with a simple exercise:

As you're reading these words, become aware that you're holding this book. Bring your attention to the breath. Your breath is moving inside of your body. Where do you find it moving? Somewhere in your belly? In your chest? Or simply as the air flowing in and out through your nostrils? Take your time to notice the quality of your breathing. Is it tight, easy, deep, shallow, fast, slow?

Notice how it's possible to read and to be aware of your body breathing at the same time. Let awareness of both things be here.

Now try something: Squint your eyes as if you're trying to focus on the details of each word. Keep squinting and feel your breathing now. What's changed? Has your breath become shallow or stopped altogether? Now soften and relax the muscles around your eyes, gently opening your vision a little more to the whole page as you read. How does your breath feel different now?

This is an example of how the breath and the muscles in the body are interconnected. Your breath restricts with muscle tension and releases when muscles relax. Think about how much you probably squint your eyes when you're reading on the computer or your phone. Watch what happens when you allow yourself a nice deep breath. Your breath can lead the way, helping to release and relax the tension in your body.

WHAT IS BREATHWORK?

Breathwork is breathing consciously to support yourself physically, emotionally, psychologically, and spiritually. It broadly refers to any practice based on awareness and direct guidance of the breath. It's about intentionally changing your breathing pattern in specific ways to achieve different outcomes. What kinds of outcomes? Relaxation of the body and the mind, increased energy and vitality, emotional release and balance, and even expanded states of consciousness. Once you open up to the practice, you'll realize that it's here to support you throughout your lifetime.

If it sounds esoteric or intimidating, know that breathwork can be pretty simple. Even a 30-second breath exercise can transform the way you feel. A longer breathwork process can unwind deep tensions you've been holding for years. Breathwork can help with many health conditions—anxiety, insomnia, blood pressure, pain, fatigue—as well as any difficult emotions, such as fear or anger. Not only that, it can take you from feeling good to feeling great.

The basic principle of breathwork—and why I love working with the breath—is that it shows you, in an immediate, experiential way, how healing comes from within. Simply by breathing with conscious intention, you become aware of your power to nourish yourself and to change the way you feel at any given moment. I see this all the time as a breathwork practitioner, and this book will help you access this power you have inside.

In one form or another, breathwork has been around forever, with ancient origins in India, China, Japan, Tibet, and Greece, among other places. Many specific disciplines involve breathing in a conscious way—a vast lineage with many similarities and differences. My work pulls from a variety of traditions. Breathwork is rooted in the wisdom of our ancestors and is just as powerful and relevant today as at any time in history. Humans are humans. The breath is the breath.

Now let's take a moment to recognize why you're here. What are you curious to know about the breath? Have you been hearing about the power of breathwork? Has someone recommended that you give it a try? Did a health-care provider tell you that breathwork might help with a physical condition? Do you find yourself frequently holding your breath and noticing that it doesn't feel good? Do you have trouble sleeping? If you have thought *yes* to any of these questions or there's another reason that brought you here, then there's something for you in this book.

And you're not alone. These days, breathwork seems to be everywhere. It's increasingly referenced in popular culture, and in interviews with holistic and traditional health-care providers and spiritual seekers. Breathwork is being recognized as a critical component of self-care, a reliable and highly beneficial way of staying grounded, calm, and energized in times of stress and uncertainty. You may see breathwork mentioned on social media feeds or as part of a comprehensive wellness approach in schools or the workplace. It's often cited as an important element in recovery after strenuous exercise. In each instance, breathwork is acknowledged as a portal to mental and physical fitness and emotional well-being.

I'm going to tell you something that may seem surprising: Your breath is the most central function of the human body. You can go weeks without food and days without water but just minutes without breath. Most of us are well aware of the essential factors vital to our health and well-being such as diet, sleep, and exercise. What many don't know is that the benefits of each of these are influenced and can be greatly enhanced by the breath. For example, you may be eating healthfully, but if your breath is shallow and your belly is tight with stress, this can interfere with blood and oxygen flow into the digestive organs and the absorption of all those nutrients.

The breath also works as a powerful detoxifier; 70 percent of the toxins in your body can be released through the lungs by way of the breath. If you aren't breathing optimally, the rest of your body—namely the organs of elimination, including the lungs, kidneys, bowels, liver, skin, and lymphatic system—has to work harder to get rid of toxins.

A BIT OF BACKGROUND

My path to breathwork was deeply personal. Growing up, I often felt restricted in my breathing, the result mostly of anxiety and insecurity, especially in school. I couldn't read out loud in school because I didn't have enough breath to finish a sentence. My body was tense and my mind was blocked unless I was in motion, whether through sports or dance. Those physical activities led me to pursue teaching various types of fitness, including aerobics for ten years. Later, my study of Kundalini yoga introduced me to breathing exercises called pranayama. This is how I discovered that you could feel energy in your body from breathing intentionally. I realized that you don't have to be an athlete or a dancer or even someone who enjoys strenuous activity to access the power of breath. Anyone can experience this expansive sense of freedom.

I had my first facilitated breathwork experience in 1987, when I was guided into a circular flow of breathing, today commonly called conscious connected breathing. That means breathing without pausing between the inhale and the exhale. I was curious to explore breathing this way, but as I tried it, I began to feel my breath restrict, with tightness in my gut and chest. The facilitator encouraged me to keep breathing with the tension in order to release it, and after a while, an effortless flow of breathing started to take over. My self-perception shifted instantly. Whereas I had previously identified myself as an anxious, fearful person, I now saw that I was someone who *has* fear and anxiety at times but isn't defined by them. The difference was palpable. I went from feeling powerless to completely empowered, which illuminated for me how breathwork can expand consciousness.

In some ways, the process reminded me of learning a new dance. First you learn the steps through the counts, then you count with the music. At some point, when you're ready and your body gets it, you let go of the counting and the steps and you let the music move you. You give over to it as your mind relaxes and opens, and you're no longer inhibited or controlled by your thoughts or other distractions. You're just present. After finding that inner freedom through this connected pattern of breathing, I felt part of something bigger than just my own experience.

I spent the next five years exploring breathwork with wonderful teachers. Then, inspired to share the gift of breathwork with others, I trained to become a facilitator in conscious connected breathing. At the time, I was also practicing bodywork, including Shiatsu acupressure and Swedish-style massage. Once I began to incorporate breathwork into bodywork sessions, the effects were immediately noticeable, and powerful. My clients felt more relaxed than they had after massage alone—deeply at peace, yet energized, open, and grounded. Recognizing the breath's capacity for self-soothing and healing, I gradually shifted my practice to breathwork full-time.

Engaging the breath with mindful focus remains central to my practice, thanks in part to my training in a form of therapy called Hakomi somatic psychotherapy. It combines body-oriented techniques with verbal interventions supported by unique guiding principles (such as nonviolence and mindfulness) to invite inner exploration and create positive change. Hakomi helped me to better understand psychology and to articulate what I had noticed in breath and body patterns for so many years: how the breath is a doorway for sensing what is present in the body and a portal to personal transformation and growth.

Everything in this book and the way I approach breathwork is centered around the following principles:

- MINDFUL AWARENESS. When we bring awareness to our breath, we can engage consciously with it, notice the effects of breathwork, and come into a deeper relationship with ourselves and our lives.

- LOVING-KINDNESS. Approaching breathwork as a loving and kind gesture toward yourself directly influences the outcome and deepens the benefits of breathwork.

- ORGANIC INTELLIGENCE. There's an innate wisdom to our body/mind in that the different parts are interconnected and work as a whole system. Within this system, each of us has the ability to experience our natural inclination toward vitality, growth, and healing. Breathwork creates a space to experience our inherent wholeness.

Just as I teach others to experience the power of the breath, I look to the breath as my own teacher and guide. It flows fully and freely when I'm feeling good. My breath is easy when I'm calm. It becomes shallow and holds tightness in my gut when I'm anxious or not being compassionate toward myself. And it's always here to remind me that my emotions and thoughts don't have to be in charge. When I breathe fully and easily for a while, I open up and free any tension that may have been gripping me even a moment before.

If the pandemic years can teach us anything, it's that normalcy and certainty aren't guaranteed. This thought in itself can put us into a state of stress, so it makes sense that more people now than ever are turning to breathwork. The more you utilize conscious breathing, the more you realize the power you have within you to react differently to external forces, rather than trying to resist or overcome them.

HOW TO USE THIS BOOK

As you make your way through the pages, I encourage you to take your time, even slowing down your breath to receive and absorb the information as it's presented. The three parts of this book mirror how I structure classes and one-on-one breathwork sessions. The order of the book and the practices within each chapter are designed to help you learn to use your breath to find the calm, balance, and vitality you carry within you. This grounding presence is accessible all the time, amid everyday situations—and times of extreme difficulty.

As you continue to explore further, you'll discover how the breath serves as a bridge between your brain and your body. The emphasis here is on understanding not only *how* but *why* you breathe as you do, so that you can begin to identify your own common breathing patterns and rebalance.

What I call practices are exercises or techniques that you repeat in order to cultivate a shift. Some of the practices are subtle, to gently bring you into your relationship with your breath in a mindful way. There are practices to access relaxation and practices to energize. My objective is the same for all: to help you foster a nourishing relationship with the breath, so that you may develop an empowering habit. If you find a practice difficult or you're tightening with it, you may be pushing too hard. Allow yourself to ease up, slow down, and soften a bit more with it. It's okay if you don't "feel" it. Give your body time to catch on.

As you venture further into the book, I will encourage you to get moving! Movement with breath is important for opening the body, relieving tension, and making space for the lungs to access fuller and deeper breathing. And simply to feel good!

All of this acquired knowledge will give you the tools to incorporate breathwork into your life, making it as routine and easy as getting out of bed in the morning or brushing your teeth.

From the first prompt to become aware of the breath, on page 7, to the routine-building suggestions in the final chapter, you'll keep experimenting to find what feels good and works best for you. By the end, you'll be ready to create your own breathwork program to carry you through each day.

HOW TO BREATHE YOUR WAY THROUGH THE BOOK

I began this book by asking you to notice how you were breathing as you read the words on pages 7–8. As the book progresses and the practices become more involved, it's not always easy to read and follow the instructions at the same time. I suggest that you read through a practice a couple of times to get an idea of how to do it, then put the book down and give it a try. If anything feels complicated or overwhelming, work at your own comfortable pace until it becomes easy to go through the practice without having to read along.

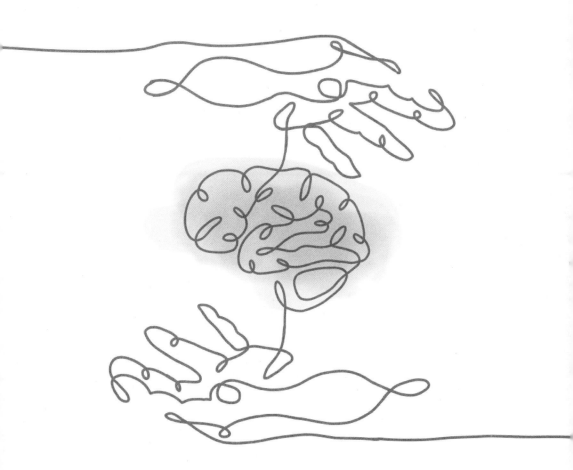

PART I

BECOMING
AWARE

One of the most beautiful gifts we receive
from breathing is the ability to perceive,
which enables us to open up a large
field of heightening our awareness.

—ILSE MIDDENDORF,
THE PERCEPTIBLE BREATH

1

Getting Familiar with the Breath

The Bridge from Unconscious to Conscious

Breath is our most intimate relationship with life. When the umbilical cord is cut at birth, we stop receiving oxygen from our mother, and we greet the world with our first inhale. We usually give a good exhale as we cry, so the lungs can inflate and begin working on their own, moving oxygen into the bloodstream and removing carbon dioxide by breathing out. Here we begin a breathing life! Breath *is* life. Our whole body, every cell, is inhaling and exhaling. This movement of life is happening within you, by most estimates, more than twenty thousand times each day.

Breath is conscious and unconscious, voluntary and involuntary. Because of its direct connection with the nervous system and the brain, breathing affects and is affected by emotions and thought patterns. That's right—even one thought can change the way you're breathing. Next time you have an upsetting feeling, notice what happens with your breathing. Does it feel tight? In contrast, next time you have a good feeling, notice your breathing. Is it more open? It's one thing to have an intellectual understanding of this connection but quite another to experience it as the movement of life happening within you, in real time, all the time. Think of the last time you sighed, yawned, laughed, cried, or yelled. Each of those actions is a way of breathing, a physical or emotional response to a variety of stimuli. By learning to observe these and other ways of breathing, you begin to become aware of the breath in your body.

The suggestions and practices that follow will guide you into a conscious relationship with the breath, working your way from the first and most important step of simply noticing, to actively participating with it.

A BRIEF HISTORY OF BREATHWORK

The history of breathwork is woven into the fabric of many cultures worldwide. We know that many wellness and spiritual practices are rooted in ancient techniques and rituals originating more than 2,500 years ago. These traditions have utilized the breath for health, energy balance, and meditation, and include pranayama in yoga from India, qigong in Chinese medicine, the mindful meditation and mantra practices of Buddhism and Hinduism, and the recitation of the rosary in Christianity (as well as any steady chanting) is now seen as a beneficial form of rhythmic breathing. Breathing exercises were even found in ancient Egyptian hieroglyphs.

In the 1920s, German psychologist Wilhelm Reich brought breathwork into psychotherapy as an additional healing practice, to release tension and encourage relaxation. He believed that conscious breathing helps expand our capacity to tolerate more energy and relax our defensive "character armoring," or protective or coping responses held in place by muscle tension and restricted breathing. Reich's work influenced other therapists in the field, including German-born psychiatrist Fritz Perls and American psychotherapist Alexander Lowen, founder of bioenergetics; they and others considered breathwork a tool for psychological well-being. In the 1960s and '70s, breathwork grew popular in therapeutic practices and healing circles. Psychotherapist Leonard Orr introduced Rebirthing Breathwork, inspired by circular breathing, or conscious connected breathing, and grounded in his theory that the breath could be used to resolve birth trauma, unlock deeply held tension patterns in the unconscious mind and body, alleviate pain, and cure physical ailments. Around the same time, psychiatrist and consciousness researcher Stanislav Grof developed Holotropic Breathwork, an accelerated connected breathing method, to explore the psyche and altered states of consciousness. Several schools have evolved from these early models as a similar practice yet with a different focus and intention. Today, there are countless ways to pursue working with the breath.

TAKE A MOMENT

Notice and Observe

Notice your breathing. Does it feel tight, easy, deep, shallow? Now try clenching your jaw and clamping your teeth together. Look very carefully at the flow of your breathing. What changes do you notice? Now release and soften your jaw and unclench your teeth. Notice any changes to the flow of your breathing.

BEFRIENDING THE BREATH

Now that the breath has your attention, you begin to develop a relationship with it. Awareness is a state of consciousness that allows you to notice your breath in the present moment. Awareness is also the bridge between the conscious and unconscious. Without awareness, the breath operates strictly on an unconscious level. Noticing and accessing the breath gives you space to actively respond to any changes in it.

Most of the time, you go about your day largely unaware of your breath and its constant activity. When you run into circumstances that cause your breathing to change or become irregular, your brain shifts into another gear; your chest may get tight, and your emotions may heighten. Your breathing may soon feel off-kilter and shallow. The way forward is to recognize it and intentionally change the way you're breathing. And it is with awareness that we can enter into a conscious relationship with our breath, the inner support for every part of ourselves.

Think about what happens when you're interested in getting to know someone new. First you're curious. Then you begin learning more about them, looking forward to seeing them, starting a conversation, wanting to talk more often, and beginning to identify their qualities and quirks. That's how we grow closer. Tensions may arise, but if the relationship is valuable to you, you work it out. This is someone to turn to whenever you need them, unconditionally, 24/7.

Now imagine this "someone" is your breath. Always here, with you and for you. Right now, feel it within you. Just by looking for the movement of your breathing, you're coming into a conscious relationship with it while also bringing yourself deeper into your body and out of your busy mind. What you find is secondary to simply looking for and feeling it. Once you give the breath attention, you're more connected to every part of yourself—your body, emotions, mind, state of consciousness, and spirit. The breath will inform and guide you. It knows where to go and what to do. You can learn to trust it. To start, spend some time getting to know it.

TAKE A MOMENT

Be Curious

Close your eyes and bring your attention to your body, breathing for 5 breaths while you find and feel the rhythmic movement of your breathing, no matter how big or small, comfortable or uncomfortable. As you experience how breathing feels in your body, acknowledge anything that comes to you—thoughts, sensations, feelings. Take 5 more breaths. You just stepped into relationship with your breath. Spend more time there. Notice what happens.

THE WISDOM OF THE BREATH

The innate wisdom of the breath is perhaps our greatest natural resource. When you observe the breath along with conscious breathing, you begin to experience its interconnection with the body, how

The innate wisdom of the breath is perhaps our greatest natural resource.

you feel, and the nervous system, which includes the brain. Allowing the exhale to fall freely is how we are designed to breathe when we are in a relaxed state. It reminds our bodies to experience the freedom of being, without forcing, holding, or pushing. This invites the inhale to flow in with ease, providing us with energy and vitality. Trust the wisdom of this natural design as you allow your breath to open and flow freely. The result is the ability to actively respond to your body's tensions, to feel grounded, and to more easily find a calm and balanced state, regardless of any changes around you.

Feel the life force of the breath.

On your next exhale, let the air flow out, and wait patiently for the inhale to come on its own. Take your time—don't rush it. The key is to wait. Feel the force or impulse that makes you want to inhale, and then receive it. Repeat. Let the exhale fall, then wait, keeping your attention still and present. Don't try to hold the breath out (but even if you did, no matter how long you try, at some point, this life force energy, or prana, will make you inhale and take it in). As you stay with this exploration a couple more times, see what it's like to be conscious of how your body wants you to breathe. Is it simply the unconscious impulse of your body balancing the gas exchange of oxygen and carbon dioxide, telling a bunch of neurons in the base of your brain to make you breathe? Or is it the life force energy that makes you breathe? Both. The oxygen is the vehicle, and the breath energy (prana) is the effect. Becoming aware of this energy brings an understanding that life wants you to breathe. Feel this awareness at least once a day—or all day!

Breathwork can unlock parts of you that you didn't know were closed. Nia took my breathwork class online in 2020 during the COVID-19 pandemic lockdown, a stressful time for all of us. In the hour-long class, I led her through practices to wake up awareness of the breath in the body, movement practices to open the breathing spaces, and, finally, a 10-minute connected breath session during which Nia was lying down. At the end of the class, she felt deeply relaxed. The next day, she called to let me know she had dreamed that night, which was very significant for her. She explained that her father, a psychologist who studied dream interpretation, had died in 2018. Nia had loved to spend time with him talking about the many dreams she had had through the years. After his death, she had stopped dreaming—until the night after that breathwork class. Losing her father at a fairly young age was traumatic for her, and it was her body's wisdom that closed off that place in her unconscious until she felt secure enough to reopen it herself. She was so relieved, and a bit surprised that a class on breath could allow that to happen. I can be surprised when experiences like this happen, but I'm never shocked, because I trust the wisdom of the breath to open the deeper places within us when it feels safe.

BREATH AWARENESS PRACTICES

The following practices are designed to raise your awareness of the breath. Though there is no one universal way to breathe, there are optimal ways to approach breathwork. Curiosity keeps us from dwelling in our critical, skeptical minds, encouraging us instead to remain open-minded, present, and receptive. As a result, we develop a more expansive perspective, which helps us learn new things and change for the better.

PRACTICE
Take Your Seat

This practice involves scanning your body as you become aware of the breath. As you turn your attention to each area, imagine you're walking into your own house, going from room to room and noticing what's before you, just as it is.

» Sit comfortably and become aware of the solidness that supports your body. Feel your feet on the floor or whatever they are touching. Give your feet to the ground. (You don't have to be taught how to do that; just see what your body does.)

» Feel where your seat is touching the chair or surface you're sitting on, and give in to that surface.

» Slowly scan for any sensations or energy in your body: warm, cool, tight, soft, buzzing, tingling, tired, heavy, light, numb, alert—whatever feeling comes to you. Just take notice, without doing anything.

» Now check in with how you're feeling. Notice any emotion, and sit with it for a moment. Can you stay curious without evaluating it?

» Now become aware of the air flowing in and out of your nose. Is it warm or cool? As you inhale, follow the air in through your nose and down into your body. Is there a place in your body where you can feel the movement of your inhale? As you exhale, also notice what moves. Feel where that movement is happening without trying to alter it. It might change just by you noticing it. Be curious about the places where you can feel your breathing. Do you find it somewhere high in your chest area? Or in your abdominal area? Or somewhere between in your solar plexus and your lower rib cage? Your back? Your pelvis and hip area? Throat? More than one place? If it's hard to feel your breathing, that's okay. Notice how (and where) you're aware of the inflow and outflow.

» When you find the movement of your breath, put your hand on that area. If it's in more than one place or it feels spread all over, put your hand on the place that's moving the most or that you're drawn to. Be here, feeling the contact of your hand on your body and the movement of the breath in your body under your hand.

» Feel the rhythm as your body moves one way on the inhale and another on the exhale. Imagine that right in the middle of that movement is a big comfy chair that you can sink into, and let yourself rest in the center of the flow of energy that nourishes you as you feel your breathing coming and going.

» Now relax your hands in your lap and stay here, simply observing the rising and falling of your breath as it moves within you. It's natural for your mind to wander. When you catch it drifting, try to bring it back to your breathing. You can do just this for a few moments throughout the day. As you practice this, over time, notice how your overall awareness of the breath grows. Let the wisdom of your breath do what it knows how to do. Rest here.

PRACTICE
Discovering Your Breathing Spaces

This practice brings awareness to the spaces where the breath is in motion within your body, so that you can get acquainted with and feel the potential and full movement of respiration. Give yourself time to remain in each area until you become aware of what is happening— whether you're breathing there or not. Throughout the practice, observe with the intention of not changing the breath.

» Sit or lie down comfortably. Turn your attention to your lower abdomen, the area from your navel to your pubic bone and into your pelvis. As your breath moves naturally, notice the space inside, between your belly and lower back. What do you notice within? Is it open? Soft? Tight? Numb? Something else? Without making anything happen, do you find your breath moving in this area?

» Bring your attention to the lower rib cage, where your solar plexus is. What do you notice right in the middle there, and in the space inside your lower rib cage area and mid back? Does your breath move inside your ribs, or is it still? Tight? Open? Something else?

» Bring your attention to your chest, your upper rib cage, and inside between your chest and upper back. Is there movement here as your body breathes just as it is? Does your chest move as you inhale or exhale, or both, or neither? Anything else?

» Bring your attention to the space inside your throat. As the air flows through your throat, what do you notice? Does it feel open, as wide as your neck, or more narrow, like a thin straw?

» As you breathe, notice each area, how it feels and any feelings or sensations that might be there. Notice the quality of your breathing—tight, easy, deep, shallow, fast, slow. Just notice how you feel in this moment after going through all your breathing spaces.

» Let's try an experiment. As you feel the air flowing through your throat and in your body, clench your jaw and notice the flow of your breath. Release and soften your jaw and notice your breathing. Now tighten your shoulders, lift them about half an inch (1.25 centimeters), and notice what happens to your breath. Let the shoulders go and notice your breathing. Now tighten your bottom and notice what happens to your breathing. Let it go and take note.

» Rest and feel what you feel. Let your breathing move however and wherever it wants, and see what that's like. Stay with that a minute and then carry on.

When Focusing on the Breath Is Uncomfortable

It's not always comfortable to focus on breathing. Since the breath is connected to the part of the nervous system that processes stress and survival (more on that in chapter 2), when we are anxious, overwhelmed, or traumatized, we will innately hold our breath. In this case, it's not the breath that people fear but the feelings or emotions held under the discomfort of their tight or shallow breathing.

I see this with some clients. As soon as they start to focus on their breath, they feel like they just can't get enough air, and they want to give up immediately. Others feel anxiety when they turn their attention to their breathing, yet they're still willing to try it. Those who have a desire to work with it can experience a powerful shift in their association with their breath, as long as it's done in a gentle, safe, and mindful way. Their body just needed to remember that breathing can feel good. (In extreme cases, when it's clear that someone feels too overwhelmed to work with the breath, I will recommend extra support from a trauma specialist.)

Easing into Your Breath

As your relationship with the breath becomes more enjoyable, it can be a source of support when you're struggling with uncomfortable feelings, whether physical or emotional. If putting all your attention on your breath creates some anxiety, however, start with a calming practice like this one.

» Turn your attention inward (close your eyes, if you like). Scan through your body and find the most comfortable, calm, quiet, peaceful place inside, without tension or "noise." It could be anywhere in your torso, your limbs, your head, a finger, an elbow, an earlobe—it's there somewhere. Take your time.

» When you find it, feel it, sink into it like when you find that perfect spot in your bed at night and can finally rest. What made you choose this place? What tells you this is a comfortable spot? Is it void of sensation? Is it warm, still, soft, spacious, quiet, or something else?

» Settle there and hold the awareness for a moment. Then feel your breath moving in and moving out. Imagine your inhale is like a little stream and let it find its way to this comfortable spot, creating space for it.

» Now imagine that your exhale can carry and spread this feeling slowly throughout your body. Inhale, giving it space; exhale and let it spread. Breathe in an easy flow to freely carry the comfort in any direction it wants to go. Keep going until it has spread to every part of your body, to every cell.

» Rest there in your comfortable space for 3 to 10 minutes or as long as you want. Notice how you feel now, compared to before doing this exercise.

Note: If you have trouble finding this comfortable spot inside, look for something that appeals to one of your senses and gives you comfort—the smell of an essential oil or flower, your pet's soft fur, or the sound of soothing music. Notice how good this feels, then follow the practice above to let your breath carry that feeling throughout your body.

A Breathing Moment with My Mom

My breathwork practice is grounded in a compassionate approach, meaning I consider our self-protective instincts to be innocent. Our natural responses are the result of conditioned, habitual patterns. With any new client, I begin by gently approaching any fear with the spacious and calming resource that the breath can be. Bringing gentle breathing into the mix, with guidance at first, reconnects us with the good feelings of the natural energy flow in our bodies. Directing kindness toward the discomfort begins to replace fear with a sense of ease and safety.

In the early 1990s, when I was just beginning my breathwork practice, I went home to visit my parents. To my great surprise, my mom, a heavy smoker and one of the most anxious people I've known, agreed to try a session. I could tell she was a bit uncomfortable, and yet as I write this, I am touched by the memory of her willingness to lie down and follow my guidance. Before the session was halfway through, her panic presented itself. She declared that she had had enough, then jumped up and lit a cigarette. Smoking was her way to self-soothe, and she felt vulnerable without a cigarette in her hand and breathing in that familiar way. I watched her inhale deeply, as if trying to suck in enough smoke to envelop her fear, then flicker her eyelids as she exhaled, as if to push the fear as far away as possible.

In those days, my breathwork practice involved faster-paced breathing. I wasn't experienced enough to recognize the signs that I needed to help my mother slow down and modulate the breathing process. I didn't know how to work with her in a gentle way, or even to just acknowledge her bravery in vocalizing when it was time to stop. After I became certified in Hakomi somatic psychology (see page 13), I learned more about the nervous system, which helped me understand the connection between breathing and emotions.

I now see that she was retreating to the same pattern she had followed for years in an effort to stay calm and in control of her feelings. However unhealthy, smoking was my mother's resource for comfort and relaxation because she didn't have another way to release the tension her body held. It was her survival response. She needed support, not pushing, which was her breathing habit from blowing the smoke out so many times a day. If I were working with her today, I would move slower to guide her through the breathing gently and help her settle, while recognizing her beautiful heart, innocence, deep soul, and bright spirit.

HANDS-ON BREATH AWARENESS

As another way to heighten awareness, your hands can help you stay connected to your body and sense how your body is breathing.

At some point in my breathwork sessions, I ask clients to lie on the massage table in my office and then guide them through a connected flow of breathing. I use my hands to contact the breathing areas and help my clients feel their body move and open with their breath and the natural flow of inhaling and exhaling. When the COVID-19 pandemic struck in 2020, I began holding sessions and classes online. This disconnected me physically from my clients, and I didn't know how effective this new way of working would be. The unexpected gift was realizing the natural power that people possess to connect and deepen their relationship with their breath by using their own hands to feel and direct the breath to specific areas of the body to offer a soothing salve for tension.

Awareness and Interoception

Awareness is not just important for noticing the breath but also necessary for taking action and becoming more conscious of yourself overall. That's why awareness is the core of many meditation practices. When we're mindful of our breath, we can be more connected to what the body is communicating through gut feelings, emotions, and sensations such as hunger, fullness, and heartbeat. This kind of inner awareness, known as "interoception," allows us to recognize and therefore better regulate our emotions, manage stress, and tend to myriad needs. Awareness is the first step in creating change in our lives. Your breath is the best doorway for welcoming the change in.

Wake Awareness with a Rub

This practice can be energizing and grounding, and is an excellent way to start your day or feel your flow of breathing at any time.

» Place your hands on your lower abdomen, between the navel and the pubic bone, and rub in a circle up the right side and down the left a few times. Feel the warmth of your hands as you gently rub your belly.

» Now hold your hands still over that area and let your breath find its way under your hands like a stream or a light breeze. Take a few breaths. Wait until you feel soft and easy movement of your breath under your hands.

» Then move your hands to your solar plexus or lower rib cage and repeat the circle with your hands over this area for as long as it feels good.

» Hold your hands still here and let your breath find its way under your hands.

» Next, put your hands on the sides of your ribs and rub up and down vigorously but comfortably. This fast rubbing can stimulate and loosen your breathing muscles (more about those in chapter 2) and energize you.

» Now hold your hands still on the sides of your ribs and let your breath gently find its way inside your hands for a few breaths.

» Bring your hands to your chest. Repeat the circular rubbing (or rub in any direction that feels good) a few times, then hold your hands there, letting your breath make its way under your hands.

» Rub your lower back up and down vigorously a few times, then hold your hands there. Notice any subtle movement of your breath under your hands. Stay there for a few breaths. We don't usually think about breathing here, but your back is also part of the movement of respiration.

» Now, with your fingertips, softly stroke your throat downward. Feel the contact and sigh a few times as you stroke.

» Hold your hands over your throat and feel your breath slowly flowing through your throat.

» Now let your hands go to any part of your body that could use attention, comfort, loosening or energizing as you gently breathe.

» Rest for a moment and notice how your body feels and how your breathing is flowing. Is it easier for your breath to find these places in your body after that contact?

*Sit and rest
in the place*

where your breath comes and goes.

Giving In to Gravity

Giving your body and breath to gravity is a great awareness practice. We spend so much time "doing" in our lives that we can easily forget how to "not do." Awareness practices can help us undo this habit so we can feel what it's like to just be. Giving your body to gravity means letting go without trying to let go. Giving your breath to gravity means giving in to the downward out flow of the air and letting your muscles soften with it. This can help your breath and body find ease and is an important first step to beginning any conscious breathing practice. When we're stressed, our bodies resist the downward pull and grounding support of gravity, as we are holding on and not letting go. Our muscles can tense up, our shoulders may rise, and we feel the air not leaving our lungs adequately and freely.

Explore the effects for yourself: Exhale only halfway and then try to take a full, free inhale. Notice what that's like. Try this a few times in a row, and you will begin to understand how tension builds in your body. Holding in the breath like this often means stiffening the body, with a habitually tight chest that has forgotten how to soften and move downward with the out breath. Giving in to gravity feels like dropping in or settling down. Our body knows the direction of calm and relaxation even if we aren't conscious of it.

Grounding with Gravity

This practice brings awareness to the power of gravity and stability to release tension patterns and, in turn, the exhale. Imagine you vigorously shook a snow globe and are watching the snow falling inside. As those little flakes float downward, making their way to the bottom, connect your exhale to their motion. Let your breath fall softly with them, slow and easy, taking all the time it needs, no rush. Let your shoulders and your jaw fall as a downward release. It's a free fall, not a pushing out. Your breath might be long, or it might be short at first. That doesn't matter, because with repetition, your body begins to get the hang of it and the breath continues to lengthen with each exhale. Now rest for a moment, noticing any way you feel different in your body. Let the support of gravity, of the ground, hold you—every muscle, bone, and organ. Rest here for as long as you want.

After a session, it's very common for a client to say, "I feel heavy but light at the same time. I feel connected to myself!" That's the sensation of being grounded and present yet free, a result of fatigue falling away. I've also witnessed many people tearing up as they release the breath, finally letting go of the tightness of long-held emotions and allowing more space for the inhale to expand.

Sheila hoped that breathwork would provide some relief from the fear and stress she felt in her relationships. Her breath was very tight and shallow. She could hardly inhale, and tightened her lips to exhale. She was afraid to open up and let go. I guided her to notice her breath as it was in that moment and then practiced gently giving more space for the exhale to fall. A few breaths were all she could handle before she started listing all her problems. Still willing, she lay on the table and learned to breathe in a gentle, connected flow.

As I made contact with her breathing spaces with my hand, her chest and ribs began to soften as she breathed out.

Allowing her exhale to fall freely helped relax the tightness, and she learned to soften into her vulnerability. She left each session with a kinder attitude and determination to return and practice. After a few months, her breath became easier to access, her compassion for herself and others increased, and she had a more tolerant view of the world around her. She learned how even a little breathing could shift her out of a heightened state of stress. One of the most compelling things about facilitating breathwork with clients is their shift to a more open perspective and a newfound trust in the wisdom of the breath.

*Awareness
is the
first step
in creating
change.*

Your body is your first home.
Breathing in, I arrive in my body.
Breathing out, I am home.

—THICH NHAT HANH

2

Connecting Body, Brain, and Breath

An Integrated Intelligence

We are born knowing the natural freedom of breathing. Newborns make the heroic transition from water to air as their source of oxygen moves from the umbilical cord to the lungs. The respiratory system continues to develop throughout childhood, especially in the first two to three years. The lungs grow, adapt, and fill, and the abdomen and rib cage begin to gently expand. As we grow older and begin to experience the challenges of life, however, we unconsciously learn to breathe shallowly. We tighten our bodies and hold our breath when we feel unsafe or uncertain. Thanks to the design of our nervous system, however, we can learn to consciously use our breath, deliberately lengthening and pacing it in order to manage difficult or threatening circumstances and help our body remember our natural free breath.

The human body is a dynamic system, capable of bouncing back from difficult experiences. Our inherent capacity for resilience is seen in the body's ability to move through challenges and to heal. Breathing is instrumental in developing this ability to shift from a stressed state to a calm one on a regular basis. In its natural and balanced state, our breathing is meant to be fluid and responsive, adaptive and free rather than controlled all the time.

Clearly, the breath is a powerful life force. The way we breathe influences the functions of the body and brain that, in turn, impact our experience of living. Understanding those connections, and in particular how the breath interacts with the nervous system, is another essential component of awareness. Exploring the breathing muscles is also crucial, so that we may learn to free them and create more ease and inner space.

BREATHING BY DESIGN

Day to day, you don't have to think much, if at all, about breathing. In fact, you have been breathing the whole time you have been reading this perhaps without even noticing. That's because respiration is a function of your autonomic nervous system (ANS), part of the larger, more comprehensive nervous system. The nervous system is made up of two parts: the central nervous system (your brain and spinal cord) and the peripheral nervous system (the nerves that branch out from the central nervous system to every part of your body). Your ANS is part of the peripheral nervous system. Remembering these names can be confusing, but for the purpose of understanding the breath, let's focus on the ANS. As you sit quietly, the ANS functions involuntarily to keep you going. It influences basic, and critical, bodily functions—your heart rate, breath rate, digestion, blood pressure, and body temperature regulation, to name a few—all without conscious thought on your part. This crucial branch of your nervous system is located in the brain stem, the oldest area of the brain, also known as the primitive brain, which we share with all animals, including reptiles (hence why this is sometimes called the "lizard brain"). The ANS also controls our instincts for survival and self-preservation, helping us assess when we feel safe or threatened.

To picture how these responses developed, it helps to imagine the earliest humans gauging the safety of their surroundings. These responses have remained largely the same from prehistoric times up to the present.

Here's where it's relevant to breathwork: The ANS is divided into two main branches—the sympathetic nervous system (SNS) and the parasympathetic nervous system (PNS)—each of which affects, and is affected by, the quality of our breathing. The distinction between the two branches is that the SNS is the excitation or arousal branch, activated each time you inhale (or breathe faster), while the PNS controls the body at rest, the relaxation response, and is triggered when you exhale (or breathe slower). If you're stressed or scared, the inhale speeds up automatically, and if you want more energy, you can inhale deeper and faster intentionally, both turning on the SNS to different degrees. Think of it in this simple way:

Inhale to energize.
Exhale to relax.

The key to healthy regulation of the breath—and, in turn, the brain and body—comes in knowing when and how to consciously influence the ANS. Once you understand its two-part structure (the SNS and PNS), you can learn to regulate your body and mind, including calming physiological responses like a racing heart rate or clenched muscles when you're nervous or anxious.

AUTONOMIC
NERVOUS SYSTEM

PARASYMPATHETIC | SYMPATHETIC
NERVOUS SYSTEM | NERVOUS SYSTEM

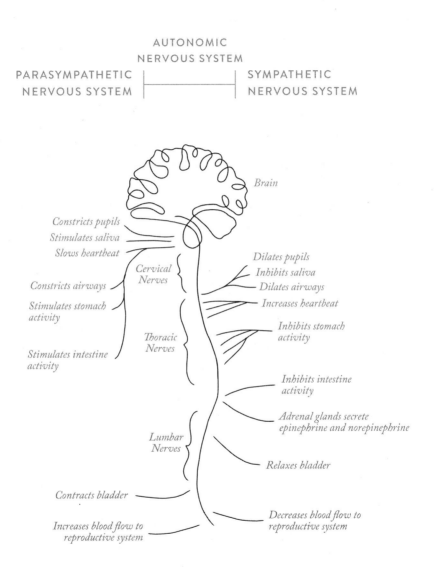

Brain

Constricts pupils
Stimulates saliva
Slows heartbeat

Dilates pupils
Inhibits saliva
Dilates airways
Increases heartbeat

Cervical
Nerves

Constricts airways

Stimulates stomach
activity

Inhibits stomach
activity

Thoracic
Nerves

Stimulates intestine
activity

Inhibits intestine
activity

Adrenal glands secrete
epinephrine and norepinephrine

Lumbar
Nerves

Relaxes bladder

Contracts bladder

Increases blood flow to
reproductive system

Decreases blood flow to
reproductive system

When the ANS is in balance, you are alert, active yet calm, and generally feeling good. Picture your body when you feel truly at ease. Your shoulders are relaxed, and your breath is low and slow, originating from the belly and making its way up through your torso. This is your PNS response, when your heart rate naturally slows down, inflammation lowers, and blood pressure normalizes. The body is in heal-and-repair mode, or "rest and digest," rather than the activated, excited fight-or-flight mode of the SNS. It calms the amygdala, the emotional processing part of the brain, which helps us to access the prefrontal cortex—your rational brain, which helps you think clearly, make decisions, and solve problems. Our ability to have compassion for and more easily connect with others is associated with the PNS response as well. In a threatening situation, the PNS also governs the freeze response, working to shut everything down and putting the brakes on the fight-or-flight response. This allows the body to stay still and safe when it's impossible to fight or retreat; think of the way an animal might play dead in the face of a predator.

The respiratory system is not only controlled by the ANS but can also direct it. By slowing our breathing and extending the exhale, we can "let it all out." The PNS is activated, we settle back down, and relaxation flows through the body.

THE STRESS CYCLE

There's a positive side to stress. It can connect us to our survival instincts, give us energy to take action and handle challenges, prompt us to pay more attention and stay alert, and stretch us to grow. Our nervous system is moving through the SNS and PNS organically to different degrees multiple times a day. The difficulty comes when we cannot settle down and are stuck in stress mode. Before you can use your breathing to support yourself, you need the awareness to recognize that your body has been hijacked by the stress cycle.

When our breath is restricted for any number of reasons, we experience shallow, tight chest breathing, which prevents us from taking in the optimal amount of oxygen. Via the nervous system, the brain registers that we are not getting enough air. This turns on the stress response (fight or flight). Our health is negatively impacted, leading to muscle tension and the releasing of stress hormones (adrenaline and cortisol) into our system. This affects our quality of thinking, which becomes focused on stressors such as worry, fear, or judgment. The response is more shallow chest breathing and less airflow in the lungs, and the continuation of the stress cycle.

The diagram of the stress cycle on the following page is designed to help you see where you are and catch yourself, so you can interrupt it as needed. Reflect on where you tend to get stuck and how it feels.

Meet the stress head-on with slow, easy breathing, and you can reverse the cycle and access a balanced, peaceful state. When you're

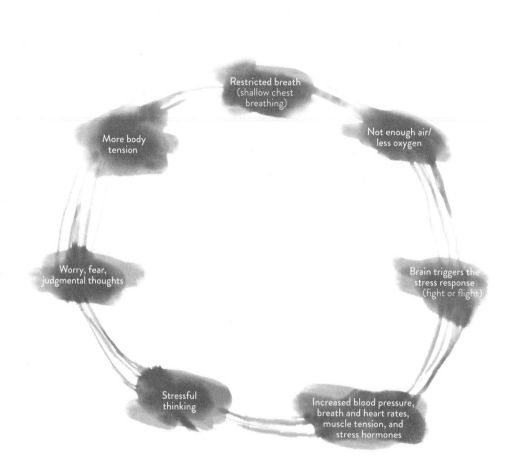

Restricted breath
(shallow chest
breathing)

Not enough air/
less oxygen

More body
tension

Brain triggers the
stress response
(fight or flight)

Worry, fear,
judgmental thoughts

Increased blood pressure,
breath and heart rates,
muscle tension, and
stress hormones

Stressful
thinking

stuck in the stress cycle, the priority is to tend to your body, not your mind. It's not the time to make a decision or figure things out. When the breath is tangled up in the stress cycle, breathing is the *only* system in the cycle that can also be conscious and get you off the hamster wheel.

Explore a Breath Cycle with a Yawn

Use this mini practice when you find yourself holding your breath. It's a good reminder of the fullness of a breath cycle (see the following page). Stretching with a yawn allows your breathing muscles to make more space for your lungs. This is what your body does to balance the flow of oxygen and carbon dioxide. This exercise does the same thing, letting your breath naturally and gently flow after opening it up.

» Find where the breath is moving inside you now. What is its quality? Tight, easy, deep, shallow? Whatever position your body is in, engage with that place in the back of your throat that opens when you yawn.

» Now slowly stretch and yawn as wide as you can. Feel your body and breath opening as much as feels good. At the end of the yawn, feel how your breath lets go to fall back into place. Notice how you feel after that. Try it again, but this time hold at the top of the stretch and yawn for about 3 seconds. Let it go the same as before, and take note of your breathing. Are the movement and quality of your breath different in any way, even subtly? Notice how your inhale opens with the yawn, bringing in more energy, and your exhale lets that energy settle. This completion of the circle—an easy expansion of the in breath and the free letting go of the out breath—can simultaneously ground, relax, and reenergize you. Notice how it feels counterintuitive to make a big stretch with the exhale. Your body is intelligent and, in one way or another, is always moving toward balance. The next time your body wants to yawn, luxuriate in it.

THE BREATH CYCLE

"Take a deep breath." Have you ever considered what that actually means? One way to think about it is to imagine the vastness of the ocean. Consider its depth, rather than the breadth of its surface, and try to conjure an image of how far down it is to the ocean floor. The process of breathing within the body is similar. The freer the breathing muscles and the softer the belly, the deeper the breath goes into your lower lungs, where much more oxygenated blood can be circulated. So a deep breath is not a big, fast breath as so many of us think but rather a low, expansive breath.

Taking a deep breath means more than just inhaling, however. That's only half the equation. One breath is one full cycle—the inhale *and* the exhale. For the nervous system to be in balance, there must be an easy, unrestricted flow between the in breath and the out breath. This allows the nervous system to function in an optimal state.

THE VAGUS NERVE

What if you were told about an app that would calm you down, increase your energy, clarify your thinking, release tightness in your muscles, help you sleep, decrease inflammation, strengthen your immune system, give you a youthful glow, increase your capacity for kindness, and shift your mind to a state of contentment with each

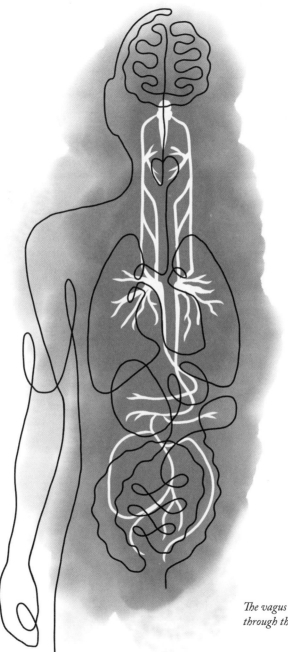

The vagus nerve branches through the body.

use? Wouldn't you jump at the chance to download it? The best part about this app is that it exists inside your body, and you can turn it on with your breath. It's called the vagus nerve, and by stimulating it, you can breathe easy, restore balance, and handle emotional, mental, and physical responses in a more centered way.

The vagus nerve has been called the key to well-being, the secret weapon in alleviating stress, and the literal mind-body connection. It's also been called the soul nerve, the love nerve, the caretaking nerve, the healing nerve, and the "wandering nerve" since it branches throughout the torso. It's also your inner switch to help you go from flipping out to chilling out. It is the longest and most complex of the cranial nerves, which originate in the brain stem. The vagus is actually two nerves stretching above and below the diaphragm and extending to the structures used for breathing, including the airway in your throat and through your diaphragm. (This helps explain why breathing accesses the vagus nerve.) Its main purpose as command central of the PNS is to deliver messages from the body (including the digestive system, stomach, intestines, liver, pancreas, and spleen) and major organs (notably, the heart and lungs) to the brain (about 80 percent); and then from the brain to the body (about 20 percent). Depending on the message—either "I'm in danger" or "I'm safe"—it helps to regulate our system.

As the vagus nerve meanders through the neck, throat, thorax, diaphragm, and abdomen, its fibers communicate to the brain about how you're breathing: fast and hard, for example, or long and slow—in other words, stressed or relaxed. That information, in turn, regulates your body's basic functions. The vagus nerve's sensory fibers help you feel your gut clench when you're anxious and afraid, a lump rise in your throat when you're emotional, your voice go shaky when you're nervous, or that celebrated buzzy sensation in your chest when you feel love.

Learning to actively stimulate the vagus nerve gives us an internal resource to rebalance and support ourselves even in the face of chaos. One of the best ways to trigger the vagus is through slow, deep, rhythmic, diaphragmatic breathing, and by lengthening the exhale.

Your vagus nerve senses that and sends a message back to the brain that all is well. We can then cultivate resilience and allow ourselves to experience a wider range of emotions without getting overwhelmed or shutting down and more easily connect with others. Stanley Rosenberg, author of *Accessing the Healing Power of the Vagus Nerve*, writes that breathing diaphragmatically not only accesses the vagus nerve for calming and balancing but is also a necessary component for social engagement.

The activity of the vagus nerve is known as the vagal tone. It's a measure of how active or strong your parasympathetic response is. Like our breathing, vagal tone is connected to our heart rate in the most intimate way. Slow breath slows down the heart rate. You can assess your vagal tone by measuring your heart rate variability (HRV), or how much your heart rate varies between your inhale (when it speeds up) and your exhale (when it slows down). The more it slows down, the stronger your vagal tone. One way to monitor your HRV is to track how quickly your heart rate slows down and returns to a resting rate after you've exercised or been out of breath.

A few practices, including slow diaphragmatic breathing with an extended exhale twice as long as the inhale, can turn on the soothing magic of the vagus nerve. Other ways are humming, or using your voice in a soothing tone or way that feels good, such as singing or chanting a phrase or a single word like *om*. Holding or rubbing your body also stimulates the vagus nerve, as does moving in a gentle rocking rhythm, softening your eyes and opening your peripheral vision, laughing, gargling, and splashing your face with or immersing your whole body in cold water.

Discover your vagal tone.

To measure your HRV, begin by finding your pulse on your wrist. (You can also buy a monitor, or use an app on a smartwatch, to find and keep track of your HRV.) Feel your heartbeat, then inhale and exhale 5 to 10 times. As you inhale, notice if you can feel your heartbeat speed up. Now exhale slowly and notice if you can feel your heartbeat slow down. Stay with it and keep noticing as you repeat this a few more times. If you don't notice any or much change between the two, your vagus nerve (and PNS) could use more attention. The practices in this chapter, including Hum and a Hug (page 64) and Freeing the Exhale (page 72), will help.

Free your exhale and your inhale will fill you. Slower. Fuller. Freer.

Hum and a Hug

Both hugging and humming stimulate the vagus nerve, for calming, grounding, and support. The following diaphragmatic breath practice brings awareness to the brain-body-breath connection, teaching you to access the relaxation part of your nervous system. It helps extend the exhale and feel the movement of your breath inside your belly and rib cage.

» Breathing through your nose, wrap your arms around the middle of your body, placing your hands against your rib cage on either side.

» Feel the hug, the warmth of your hands, and the contact of your forearms against your abdomen. Breathe naturally a few times as you direct the movement of your breath inside your ribs and abdomen under your hands and forearms.

» Now put the hand of the upper arm on your chest and keep the bottom arm around your ribs. On your next exhale, hum (use a medium or low tone), sensing the vibration of your voice inside your rib cage until the air is all the way out without straining. Allow your chest, ribs, and abdomen to soften inward as you hum the breath out.

» Feel the vibration of your voice in your body, and imagine your hum is massaging your throat and all the nerves and organs in your body.

» Wait for the inhale to come, then let it in and luxuriate in the space it's giving you. Feel the expansion of your belly under your bottom arm and ribs and gently up into the chest as you take in as much air as feels good.

» Exhale and hum the air all the way out. Imagine and feel how the sound can vibrate into every part of your body, even your head.

» Repeat 3 to 10 more times, or as many as you want to, until you feel an easy movement of expansion and softening of your belly and rib cage. This means your diaphragm has more space to move freely. Practicing this even for 3 rounds, 2 or 3 times a day, will allow you to access your relaxation response more easily.

» Relax your hands in your lap. Breathe naturally and feel what you feel. You may feel sensations in your body. Rest, then, when you're ready, begin to stretch your body in any way that feels good.

THE POWER OF THE EXHALE

Freeing the exhale allows us access to relaxation, and can simply help us breathe better. In 1965, American choral conductor and breathing specialist Carl Stough founded the Institute of Breathing Coordination, an organization that researched optimal breathing. His premise was that the exhale is the key to strengthening the diaphragm and increasing lung capacity. According to Stough, "If you can't get the exhale out, you can't get the inhale in." This may seem obvious, but it's the full exhalation that releases the stale air from the lungs and makes space for your body to receive that full and free inhale.

In his work with singers and wind instrumentalists, Stough taught them to free the diaphragm and to help it perform with more power and ease. At the VA hospital in East Orange, New Jersey, he worked with patients plagued with severe emphysema, asthma, and lung conditions with no hope of recovery. Afterward, patients were better able to let air into the lungs naturally, without the need for supplemental oxygen. Stough was later invited to coach the USA Track & Field team in the 1968 Summer Olympics in Mexico City, which resulted in a record number of gold medals. The United States was the only team that didn't need supplemental oxygen at the high altitude.

In the early 1990s, I was fortunate to watch a video of Stough at work, using vocalization on the exhale and his hands to help people soften and release the upper rib cage as they exhaled by lightly tapping and applying gentle pressure on the breathing muscles, opening the rib cage and keeping the spine flexible. The coordination of the exhale with sound and with the release of the chest ribs triggered the communication with the breathing muscles working together to create more range of motion for the diaphragm and freedom in the entire rib cage and respiratory system. When I use these practices with clients, I have found that they interrupt a pattern of shallow chest breathing and deepen breath capacity, and I watch my clients experience a feeling of relief. As they soften and let go of the chest muscles, the air flows out. They may release pent-up emotions from habitual holding, and the inhale naturally deepens without force. It's wonderful to see how good this makes them feel, every time.

Breath Sessions with Dad

One of my most powerful teaching experiences was with my father, during the last year of his life. He had been diagnosed with pulmonary fibrosis, or hardening of the lungs, making him very short of breath. An athlete all his life, he was determined to keep going, but his legs were not getting enough oxygen flow, which made it very difficult to walk. He was still living at home in California when my three siblings and I made the decision to take turns caring for him for a week at a time. I felt pretty inadequate about my caregiving skills and doubted I could handle attending to his health struggles. In the midst of all the scrambling thoughts in my head, I finally heard a voice say, *Can you take just one breath right now?* A clear, committed *Yes* bubbled up from my gut. With that one breath, I came back to my center. That question was my North Star from then on.

I wondered if Carl Stough's work with patients at the VA hospital might apply to my father's condition. Although there was no cure for pulmonary fibrosis, perhaps loosening and coordinating his breathing muscles could help. I kept noticing how tight his breath, body, and movements were, and how tense and emotionally edgy he was, clear signs that his nervous system was in stress mode. Seeing my dad this way was difficult, as I had always known him to be easygoing, energetic, funny, and optimistic.

Excited to experiment, I guided him to gently extend his exhale, whispering *la la la la la* for as long as it could go for a few breaths. I then had him count from 1 to 10, the sound of each number riding on the air flowing out as I put my hand on his chest to help the upper ribs soften with the exhale. I wiggled his rib cage downward as he continued. His breath was so tight, he could only count to 3 at most. Yet the repetitions and the light pressure of a warm hand contacting his chest ribs began to ease his breathing. As we continued, he relaxed more, and sometimes got sleepy as the tension in his muscles began to unwind. I watched his face, mood, and temperament soften with his body. He smiled at me, letting me know it was easier to breathe. I will never forget this beautiful moment with my dad and the wonderful lesson I learned about the wisdom of breath. His lungs could not recover, but his diaphragm could still find more freedom as he could access a little more breath. Allowing the breathing muscles to soften into relationship with each other allowed his nervous system to access relaxation. This experience taught me an early breathwork lesson: Even in the midst of the most excruciating discomfort, accessing a deep, peaceful state is possible, and the breath is the gateway to that.

Inhale to energize and receive.

Exhale to relax and allow.

Freeing the Exhale

This calming practice is inspired by the work of Carl Stough. Try it when you feel rushed, anxious, or tight. It may seem counterintuitive, but see what happens when you give your exhale more time for 5 to 10 rounds of this practice. The goal is to feel more space to breathe.

» Put your hand on your chest. Feel the contact and warmth or temperature of your hand. Exhale softly out of your mouth, making an *ah* sound (like a sigh of relief) and giving it as much space to empty your lungs as you can without straining.

» Wait for the inhale to come in on its own, receiving it fully with ease, then exhale, again letting it fall out to the end of the breath with a sigh. Feel the upper ribs in your chest soften downward, under your hand, without collapsing the spine at the same time. The exhale might not feel long or satisfying at first, so give it more time and repetitions for your body to understand what you're asking it to do.

» Next, give more support (this helps if you're tense and find yourself trying to force the breath out) and add a tongue movement that sounds like *la, la, la, la, la* until the air is out, starting with your speaking voice and letting it trail off to a whisper. Find a pace that feels good to you—not too fast and not too slow. Let the sound and the tongue movement carry the exhale out. Keep feeling your chest melt under your hand as the air falls out and let your shoulders soften.

» Let the inhale come in naturally, as deep as it feels good, focusing on making space inside your rib cage to fill your lungs and keeping your abdomen soft. Repeat 10 to 20 times or until your breath is freer.

» Rest and breathe through your nose, allowing your breath to flow naturally for a few moments. Feel the space inside as your breath flows through it.

VARIATIONS

Try these options to extend the exhale.

COUNTING

» Replace each *la la la la la* with a number. Count from 1 to 10 in a comfortable rhythm, in your regular voice down to a whisper. Stop at the number that you run out of breath on. When you get to 10, if you still have more air to exhale, start at 1 again.

» Keep counting this way at a comfortable pace until all the air has been released without forcing. As you progress, take note of what number you get to. Most likely, it will extend as your breathing opens and relaxes.

» Repeat 10 to 20 times or until your breath feels more open and you're calm.

This practice, also referred to as pursed-lip breathing, helps with shortness of breath and feelings of anxiety. Its emphasis is on steady flow and sound.

» Make a wind sound through rounded lips, like you are blowing out a candle or blowing bubbles as you exhale. Hear the soft wind sound coming from inside your mouth.

» When the air is all the way out, inhale comfortably through your nose. Exhale twice as long as your inhale if possible.

» Repeat 10 or more times, or as many times as you feel comfortable with until your breath is easier. If you feel light-headed, stop, breathe in and out through your nose, and soften your belly. Rest at the end and breathe naturally.

Carlos was preparing for the Olympic track and field trials in 2000. Three days before he left, he was so anxious that he told his coach he was afraid to get on the plane. His coach contacted me to see if breathwork might help. I had two days, two hours each day, to work with him. His was the tightest abdomen I'd ever seen, the result of an established pattern of holding the muscles in his core. Carlos could run very fast, but he couldn't slow down his breathing and relax in his daily life. His body had forgotten what it was born knowing, and his running perhaps satisfied his need to express the flight part of the fight-or-flight response.

In our first session, I reminded Carlos that just as he had learned to be a great runner through training, he could train himself to breathe in a different pattern with repetition. His instinct was to work hard at this breathing process, in the same way he pushed himself in his workouts. I guided him to gently give more space for the exhale, contacting his upper chest ribs with my hand so he could physically feel them soften downward as the air emptied. This allowed more space for the inhale into his belly and lower rib cage area. Staying with an easy, steady flow of breath was helping his body recall its natural freedom and ease. I could see his belly muscles soften slightly and then tighten a bit, back and forth, as if they were figuring out how to let go—and if it was safe to do so. When his body just couldn't hold on anymore, tears came, and he cried as his breath flowed deeper. Later, Carlos admitted how good it felt to let go. As his diaphragm and other breathing muscles moved freely together, he was able to release the stored emotions. I invited him to imagine the freedom he felt when he was running as he continued to breathe. He stayed with the connected, rhythmic movement of the inhale and exhale. As it began to flow more deeply, he felt a blissful buzzy feeling throughout his body. Gone was the extreme pressure he was putting on himself. Carlos got on the plane with no stress, and though he did not make the Olympic team, he felt good about his performance. He was relieved to experience his breath moving more easily in his body. He now knew how to slow and calm himself down when he needed to.

YOUR BREATHING SPACES

Every part of us—muscles, organs, bones—is designed to move with respiration because of the coordination of the breathing muscles. Even our cells breathe, as they take in oxygen and release carbon dioxide. Picture the synchronistic play of the breathing muscles as seaweed moving underwater with the current of the ocean. The same way the seaweed flows with the rhythmic pulsing of the ocean, your breathing muscles move with the rhythmic current of your breath.

It's common to hear the phrase "breathe into your belly" (it's something I say too, when I'm trying to direct the breath to the lower lungs), but air only goes in and out of the lungs. The breathing spaces are where you can feel the areas moving within you (front to back, side to side) as you breathe: through your pelvis and lower abdomen (to the navel), upper abdomen or solar plexus, chest, throat, and nose. Think about it: You can feel air in your nose and throat, and only the "movement" of respiration throughout your torso when air flows in and out of your lungs. The energy of the breath, referred to in breathwork as life-force energy, can be felt anywhere in the body as sensations, including buzzing, tingling, and warmth as the breath opens. In the practice of yoga, this life force is known by the Sanskrit word *prana*; in traditional Chinese medicine, it's called qi (or chi). (Qigong is the practice of moving the life-force energy throughout the body with movement, breath, visualization, or meditation.)

Meet Your Lungs

The journey of air becoming breath starts when the air enters through the nose or mouth into the part of your throat called the pharynx. It then moves through the larynx (your voice box) to your trachea (or windpipe), which leads to your lungs. About 5 inches (12.5 centimeters) down from your throat, the trachea divides into the bronchial tubes, two air passages in the right and left lobes of your lungs. These tubes are lined with small hairs called cilia that move like waves and catch impurities in the air we breathe, which we can then expel from the lungs by coughing, sneezing, swallowing, or clearing the throat. The bronchial tubes branch out through your lungs into smaller bronchi and even smaller bronchioles, at the ends of which are small air sacs called alveoli. In these hundreds of millions of tiny sacs, the wondrous exchange of gases happens and oxygen enters the blood. The blood transports that life-giving oxygen to your cells, then delivers waste in the form of carbon dioxide back to your lungs to be exhaled. This exchange happens on two levels: External respiration is the act of inhaling air from the environment and exhaling carbon dioxide back out of the body, while internal respiration occurs in every cell—every cell in your body is breathing.

Breathing or ventilation is 50 percent greater at the base of the lungs than at the top. Most of the blood circulation is in the bottom third of your lungs, which supports the case that breathing lower in the lungs will give us more oxygenated blood throughout our

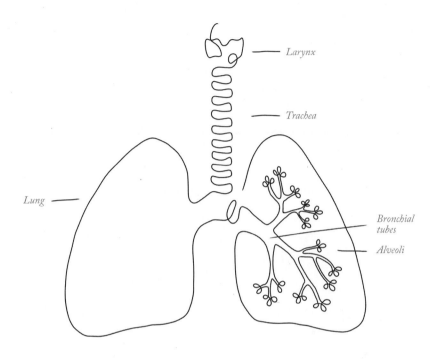

Larynx

Trachea

Lung

Bronchial
tubes

Alveoli

bodies. When the abdomen and intercostal muscles, a set of muscles between the ribs and the layers of abdominal muscles in the middle to lower part of the torso, are relaxed, the diaphragm moves freely, and you can access your lower lungs. It also slows your breathing because your body is getting enough oxygen; your lungs don't have to work as hard as they do with upper chest breathing, which uses only the upper, smaller, part of the lungs.

Nose or Mouth?

It's best to breathe through the nose for everyday breathing. Along with the gases we breathe in, such as nitrogen, oxygen, and carbon dioxide from the atmosphere, we are also exposed to an array of pollutants like dust, smog, and exhaust. A natural air purifier and filter, the nose greets these particles with cilia, the hairs that line the nasal passages. The sinuses are also lined with a mucous membrane that regulates the temperature of air as it's drawn into the body, warming, cooling, or humidifying the air, depending on what is needed. Also, air comes in slower through the nose, producing a calming, stress-relieving effect and an experience of centeredness.

We are not designed to breathe regularly through the mouth, which can create agitation by drawing air in at a faster rate. It's also less efficient, as it bypasses the mechanisms that filter and regulate the air before it reaches the lungs. In some breathwork practices, consciously directing the breath in and out through the mouth results in more expansive energy flow through the body and mind, and helps to address tension in the jaw and throat. This can be a powerfully transformative experience in conscious connected breathing (see page 12), for example. In other conscious breathwork practices, including qigong and yoga, a combination of nose and mouth breathing creates a controlled inhale and release of the exhale for body-mind balance. Regardless of the practice or process, it's important to always come back to natural breathing through the nose.

Follow the breath through your lungs.

Feel the air moving through your throat as you read this. Make a little sound like a hum right now and feel the vibration in your throat. Put a finger between your collarbones where that dent at the bottom of your throat is (the tops of your lungs are right behind these bones). Feel your breath there, where your trachea begins. Slide your fingers about 5 inches (12.5 centimeters) down from the center of your breastbone. Slide your hands apart where the trachea divides into each lobe. Rest your hands on each side of your lower rib cage and feel your lungs gently moving inside your ribs, with awareness that your alveoli are transferring gases right under your hands.

The Muscles That Breathe You

Your lungs don't pump all by themselves but rely on a group of respiratory muscles to expand with air and push it out. The principal muscle for breathing, referred to as "the diaphragm," is the respiratory or thoracic diaphragm. This big, thin, dome-shaped muscle sits within the rib cage just below the heart and lungs, separating the abdominal cavity from the thoracic (chest) cavity. Although it's a partition of the two cavities, it's a connecting force for the whole body to benefit from breath. As you inhale, the diaphragm contracts and flattens; its center moves downward and its edges move upward and out with the rib cage, creating a vacuum to pull air into the lungs. The abdomen also moves outward to make space for this to happen optimally. This is what makes belly (diaphragmatic) breathing so vital when tension has hijacked its natural movement. When you exhale, the diaphragm relaxes and moves upward, and the muscles between the ribs contract back inward, forcing air out of the lungs. It moves this way because it attaches to your sternum, inside the base of your rib cage, and to the lumbar spine. This is how the diaphragm facilitates the exchange of oxygen and carbon dioxide between the lungs and the blood essential for life.

Diaphragmatic breathing is widely reported to have a host of health benefits, including countering the effects of high blood pressure, hyperventilation, hypertension, anxiety, chronic pain, heart and gut problems, and insomnia, among other ailments, due to its powerful influence on the PNS. This muscle has several nicknames. Some call it the emotional muscle, because through the nerves that connect to it, it responds to every feeling we have. The Taoist master Mantak Chia calls it the spiritual muscle, as it can allow us to take in this sacred life force energy and bring the mind to a state of conscious awareness (prana, qi, and other ancient words for life energy also mean both breath and spirit). I like to think of the diaphragm as the space maker since it essentially creates room for your lungs to fill with and empty of 6½ quarts (about 6 liters) of air per minute, for your internal organs and lymph system to be massaged, and for your body and mind to feel an inner openness. The diaphragm is also

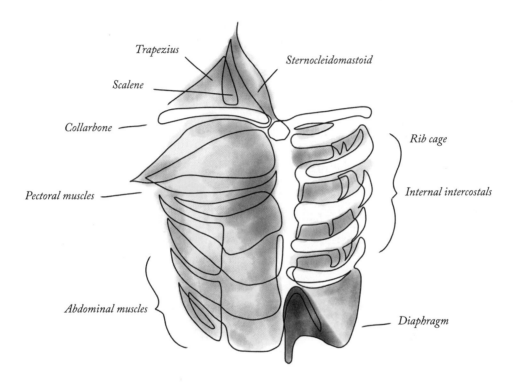

Trapezius

Sternocleidomastoid

Scalene

Collarbone —

Rib cage

Pectoral muscles —

Internal intercostals

Abdominal muscles

Diaphragm

considered the rhythm keeper, connecting to and influencing the pace of your heart as it regulates the pulsing of life within you, up to twenty-two thousand times a day.

The coordinated dance of breath movement is aided by many muscles working in sync. The pelvic floor muscles, which act as your pelvic diaphragm, subtly move in the same downward motion as the respiratory diaphragm when we inhale and relax upward as we exhale. The epiglottis, sometimes called the laryngeal diaphragm, is the flap of cartilage at the top of your trachea. It stays open for breathing and closes to keep food out. The other primary breathing muscles working to drive respiration are the intercostals and the layers of abdominal muscles in the middle to lower part of the torso. These main muscles are aided by "helper" muscles located in the upper part of the body, which work with the upper part of the lungs and support the primary muscles when respiration is in high demand—when you exercise or during an asthma attack, for example. Among these helper muscles is the chest muscle known as the pectoralis minor; the trapezius (located at the top of your shoulders); the big muscles on either side of your neck called the sternocleido-mastoids; and smaller muscles in your neck called the scalenes. A healthy regular, open breath creates a rhythmic coordination of your primary muscles moving together without the need for the work of the accessory muscles unless more effort is called for. If we are shallow chest breathing, we are only using the upper accessory muscles, which prevents the body from utilizing the stronger primary muscles and, thus, filling the lungs to capacity.

Connecting with Your Diaphragm

To feel your diaphragm, first place your fingers at the bottom edge of your rib cage on each side, about an inch (2.5 centimeters) from the center. Lightly tuck your fingers under your rib cage and hold them there for a few slow, easy breaths. Feel your lungs expanding above your diaphragm as it moves down toward your fingers, and your upper abdominal muscles pushing outward as you inhale and back in as you exhale. Close your eyes and feel the subtle movements that are happening deep inside, imagining the movement described above. Explore with your fingers from your sternum down, one breath at a time, to the bottom of each side of your rib cage. Allow your belly to soften and expand as you inhale and explore this. This can help your body remember diaphragmatic breathing.

WAKE UP THE
BREATHING MUSCLES

The next three practices are designed as a sequence. With the help of your hands and body position, the trio lays a foundation that gives you a sense of diaphragmatic breathing. At the end of the three wake-up practices, sit or lie down with your hand on your belly and breathe naturally and feel the breath moving through your torso as you inhale from the pelvis, abdomen, and rib cage, and gently into the chest. As the breath goes from the bottom of your lungs to the top, think of filling a glass with water, not only upward but outward to the sides of the glass. The practices start waking up the lower rib cage to engage the diaphragm more directly and then move to the lower spaces to encourage diaphragmatic breathing.

PRACTICE

Wake Up the Respiratory Diaphragm

Dr. Bessel van der Kolk, trauma expert and author of *The Body Keeps the Score*, promotes the importance of breathing inside the rib cage. Before he would refer a patient to a therapist, he would ask, "Are you breathing inside your rib cage? Are you living inside your rib cage?" The answer was essential in determining how present the person was in their body and whether they would be open to regulating their nervous system.

» Breathe in and out through your nose. Put your hands on each side of your lower ribs. As you breathe naturally, what do you feel inside your rib cage: Movement? No movement? Tight? Open?

» Now rub the sides of your ribs up and down vigorously for about 10 seconds and then move to the front and back rib cage to awaken sensation and warm up your outer muscles. Stop rubbing and feel the effect and sensations you've created here. Keep your hands on the sides of your ribs.

» Exhale and hold the air out and gently press your hands in, being aware that your diaphragm is moving upward, pushing the air out of your lungs. Wait for as long as you comfortably can for the impulse to inhale and then let your breath flow in freely. Feel it expand inside your rib cage under your hands, with the awareness that your diaphragm is moving downward and the edges of your ribs are moving outward. Repeat 3 times.

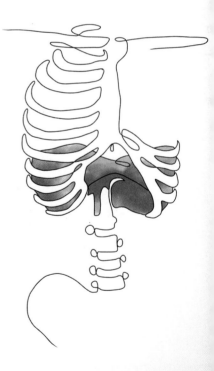

» Rest and release your hands. Breathe easy and naturally. Soften your belly and chest and continue to feel your diaphragm and ribs moving in coordination. Imagine your breath is touching the inside of your ribs. Close your eyes and stay with this for 3 to 5 minutes, sitting and breathing without forcing it.

Wake Up the Belly

Use this practice when you want to access deeper and fuller belly breathing, when you feel tight in your belly, or when you notice a sense of disconnect with your body. The amount of tension or softness in the belly will reflect how tight or free your breath is and how stressed or relaxed you feel. It can get to the point where we can't feel how tight we are holding our abdominal muscles.

» Sit in a comfortable position with your spine long and your neck soft. If your belly is very tight and it's hard to feel this area, do this lying down. Feel your back supported by the ground.

» Put your hands on your lower abdomen, on and a little below your navel. Breathe naturally and notice what you feel there under your hands. Movement? Tight? Soft? Something else?

» On your next exhale, hold your breath out and lightly press your hands into your belly as you count down from 5 to 1, then release the pressure and let the inhale fully expand as your belly softly rises without any forcing or straining. Again exhale slowly; hold your breath out and press lightly as you count down from 5. Let go of the pressure and allow the inhale to flow in, imagining a ball inside slowly and gently filling your abdominal space with air, moving outward from front to back, side to side. Repeat at least 3 more times or until you can feel the inhale filling you as your abdomen moves with ease.

» Rest and breathe easily. Keep your hands on your belly and your belly soft, and welcome your breath here, rising and falling, as you breathe deep in a steady rhythm. Give yourself 3 to 5 minutes to enjoy this, sitting or lying down and breathing naturally.

PRACTICE
Wake Up the Pelvic Diaphragm

This practice helps you feel your breath in the lower breathing space more fully, from your lower abdomen into your pelvic diaphragm. It can help you feel more grounded in and connected into your body and is a good massage for your organs.

» Sit in a chair. Feel where your bottom touches the surface of the chair. Feel the bones of your pelvis against the chair. Become aware of the movement of your breathing now as your respiratory diaphragm inside your rib cage is moving down with the inhale and up with the exhale. The pelvic diaphragm is moving with and in the same direction as your respiratory diaphragm, although it's a smaller movement and can be hard to feel, especially if there's tension in that area.

» Lean over so your chest is on your thighs, or put a pillow in your lap and lean forward onto that. Feel your belly expand out against your thigh or pillow as you inhale. As you exhale, feel your belly soften, allowing your chest and belly to drop into your thighs.

» Now think of inhaling downward into the bowl of your pelvis into the chair, and feel your pelvic floor move down a bit as your belly expands. Imagine a ball inside your pelvis expanding in all directions. Exhale and feel your body relax down into the chair.

» Continue to inhale and exhale, feeling the expansion and gentle contraction. Feel the rhythmic coordination of your belly and pelvic diaphragm working together to open your lower breathing space and invite a freer range of motion to your respiratory diaphragm as it moves with them. Stay with this for a minute or more, until you can feel the movement.

» Now sit up. Rest and breathe naturally and continue to breathe low and down toward your pelvis. Notice if you can still feel the gentle rhythmic inner movement, expanding outward and softening in. How do you feel different after this exploration?

VARIATION

Depending on what feels most comfortable and accessible to you, you may wish to try this option to wake up the pelvic diaphragm.

» Lie on your back with your knees pulled in to your chest. Breathe into the pelvic bowl in the same way as above. After about a minute of breathing this way, bring your feet to the floor with your knees bent. Rest and notice your awareness and breath moving from your belly through your rib cage and chest.

PRACTICE
Rocking Spine

Rhythmic rocking also stimulates the soothing effect of the vagus nerve. This is an adapted version of a foundational practice in Kundalini yoga called spinal flexes. The practice helps to loosen and soften your spine, inviting healthy nerve flow from bottom to top, keeping it flexible. It also opens and gently stretches the intercostal muscles of your whole rib cage, keeps your diaphragm free to keep the breath flowing, and improves circulation to your brain to help with mental clarity. Try it at least twice a day for 2 to 10 minutes, to rebalance your body for better breathing after sitting too long at the computer or looking down at your phone for long periods of time, for example.

» Sit in a chair with your hands on or above your knees or cross-legged on the floor with your hands on your shins.

» Rock forward on your sit bones as you slightly arch your back while inhaling into your abdomen and down into your pelvis, expanding your belly. Exhale and roll back toward your tailbone and sacrum as your back rounds. Let your belly and rib cage move forward as you inhale and soften back as you exhale. Rock forward, roll back, breathe in, breathe out, allowing your spine to flex forward and round backward. Your head stays centered, in line with your pelvis, and your neck and jaw stay soft and relaxed, as your neck moves naturally with the movement.

» Find a comfortable, easy, soothing rhythm of rocking and rolling back and forth as if you're your own rocking chair. After a couple of minutes, if your body wants to rock in another direction, just go with it and keep the same easy rhythm going. Let your spine and rib cage stay loose and free.

» Repeat this rocking and rolling for at least 2 minutes and up to 10 minutes (or longer, if it feels good).

» Rest and breathe naturally. Feel what you feel. Notice the sensations in your body. Is your breath more open?

PRACTICE
Stretching to Make Space

These three sitting exercises are designed as a sequence and are adapted from Donna Farhi's *The Breathing Book*. They are used to stretch the intercostal muscles between your ribs more deeply, in order to create more freedom to breathe into the lungs in the back, sides, and front of your rib cage. You can sit on the floor or a chair. If you're sitting in a chair, sit toward the front with your back away from the back of the chair. (As an alternative, you can do any of these while standing with your feet open a little wider than hip-width apart and your knees slightly bent.)

BACK

» Clasp your hands together, inhale, and stretch your arms straight up overhead. Exhale and lower your arms straight out in front of your chest and round your back.

» Inhale and feel your back expand, and then soften with the exhale.

» Take 3 to 5 long, slow, smooth breaths into your rounded back.

» Come back to a straight spine and feel the sensation of your breath gently moving your lungs and back muscles out and in.

FRONT UPPER RIBS

» Clasp your hands behind your back, stretching down and slightly away from your tailbone.

» Squeeze your shoulder blades together, stretching your arms a few inches (about 7.5 centimeters) away from your tailbone. Relax the back of your neck with your chin slightly down.

» Breathe 3 to 5 long, slow, smooth breaths into your upper ribs (chest), stretching your upper lungs under your collarbones.

» Come back to neutral, relax your arms, and gently breathe into your chest. Feel your breath moving in the space you just created inside your chest.

SIDES OF RIB CAGE

» Stretch your right arm up over your head and bend to your left side to stretch the right side of your rib cage. Put your left hand on the right ribs and rub for a moment. Hold it there and send your inhale into your hand to expand the right side of your rib cage. Exhale and feel your ribs soften.

» Repeat for 3 long, slow, smooth breaths. Come back to neutral, and repeat on the other side. Relax your arms to your sides, return to neutral and gently breathe into both sides of your rib cage.

» Rest and enjoy the effects of this practice for a moment and feel your back, front, and sides, gently moving together, out and in. Let your breath flow naturally.

Sitting Body Circles

This exercise is designed to loosen your lower back, abdomen, waist, and rib cage. It begins to move energy up through your spine and feed your nerves as it gently energizes your system.

» Feel your sit bones in the chair (or on the floor if you are sitting cross-legged) as you lengthen your spine.

» Rotate your upper body in slow circles while letting your inhale and exhale flow with the rhythm of your movement. (Imagine an old-fashioned pepper grinder—your rib cage is the handle rotating above the solid base.) For example, inhale as you circle front, and exhale as you circle back. Take your time and find a rhythm that's a comfortable, slow, and easy flow. Circle in each direction 8 to 10 times for up to a minute.

» Sit and be still; notice the effects. Let your breath flow naturally and notice how the movement of your breath through your ribs and spine feels.

To fully resolve our patterns of contraction,
we must sustain a flow of breath/energy
while committing ourselves to absolute
feeling in the present moment.

—MICHAEL SKY, *BREATHING*

3

Recognizing the Patterns

Why We Breathe the Way We Do

Once we become aware of the breath, we begin to notice our own physical sensations of breathing. What does our breath feel like in our body? Do we hold it in, or breathe in a natural, rhythmic flow? Recognizing how and why we breathe as we do helps us understand the connection of the breath to our mind and body. Whether your breathing is easy and deep or tight and shallow, it touches you on every level—physical, emotional, mental, and spiritual—though you may be unaware of how your personal breath pattern comes to be.

Our breathing patterns change unconsciously with our nervous system and with how we are feeling. When these organic ways of breathing get stifled, the breath gets restricted, interfering with the full range of movement of the diaphragm and optimal breathing.

OUR BREATH, BY DESIGN

Have you ever noticed that your body has suddenly become tense, whether it's clenching your jaw or holding your shoulders up as you try to get through a busy day? Your breath is holding on, too. Or maybe you have held your breath on purpose, to keep from crying or laughing out loud. When you finally allow yourself to let go, you experience a sense of relief in the form of a laugh, a sigh, or a good cry.

When we breathe free, our breathing muscles are unrestricted. Nothing is holding, pulling, or squeezing, and we experience a sense of ease and well-being within ourselves. We tend not to notice our breath until it becomes uncomfortable—when we struggle to take a deep breath and need to lift the shoulders to get enough air in. Breathing restrictions can be interconnected with our spinning and ruminating thoughts, which originate with the emotional or mental state we find ourselves in. These are all natural responses from our bodies.

In *My Stroke of Insight: A Brain Scientist's Personal Journey*, Dr. Jill Bolte Taylor writes, "When a person has an emotional reaction to something in their environment, there's a 90-second chemical process that happens in the body." That's the life span of an emotion. After that, any remaining response is the result of staying in that emotional loop with all the attendant thoughts around it. That's when we get caught in the stress cycle, resisting and tightening, and the anxiety hangs around longer. With awareness, Taylor explains, you can watch and feel the process as it's happening and as it goes away. This is essentially what it means to get unstuck: Consciously breathe with the uncomfortable feeling, and it brings more awareness and gives the feeling space, allowing it to move on. Hold on to a reactive thought or feeling and you unconsciously hold your breath.

When we consistently breathe more freely, we're better equipped to handle emotional ups and downs, to accept the unexpected, to be flexible, spontaneous, and resilient. We have more vitality, and are more open to emotional support, love, and compassion.

Each of us is capable of returning to that uninhibited way of breathing. Through a variety of breath practices, we can promote releasing the diaphragm and the flow of breath, and we can interrupt restrictions physically and emotionally.

Many clients come in for breathwork for one reason and leave with a wholly different experience after they recognize their patterns and are able to open the breath and relax them. Even if you're not working with a practitioner, you can learn to observe your own breath, explore your own patterns, and identify areas that want and need more breathing space.

In order to interrupt restricted patterns, first become aware of them, by noticing and feeling them; holding a caring, nonjudgmental attitude; maintaining a desire to be open, to access your natural breathing pattern; and having a willingness to let your breath and body participate in the process.

In my practice, I use the term *breath pattern* to mean a "way of breathing." Technically, a breath pattern consists of two elements:

1) The **tidal volume** is the amount of air that moves into or out of the lungs with each breath cycle and is expressed as shallow or deep breathing.

2) The **respiratory rate** (or pace) of breathing is the number of breaths a person takes per minute, and is experienced in how fast or slow the breath is moving.

A normal breathing rate for an adult at rest is 12 to 16 breaths per minute. However, the way we are breathing also includes how (quality of flow) and where we are breathing in the body (high, low, or a combination). As a practitioner, I prefer the term "natural" to "normal." Observing the breath is not about pointing out anything you're doing right or wrong but about helping the body return to its natural rhythm of breathing—the way you breathed as a young child before conditioning took hold. A natural, or unconditioned, breath is felt as a free and easy breath with the resting state and lungs fully accessible, moving and with pulsating effects within the whole body.

What I call restricted patterns of breathing have also been described as abnormal or dysfunctional breathing patterns, or breathing pattern disorders. The most common of these refer to upper chest breathing, where the diaphragm is restricted from a full, free range of motion, which results in respiration happening too fast and pushing out too much carbon dioxide. One example of this type of pattern is overbreathing, which ranges from moderate chest breathing to more extreme and forceful breath (hyperventilation). Excessive breathing like this lowers the carbon dioxide levels in the blood, upsetting the balance with oxygen and the blood pH (acid-alkaline) levels. The effects on our nervous system and emotional regulation vary from feeling moderately nervous to experiencing full-blown anxiety or panic. The restricted patterns of breathing addressed in this book have more subtle characteristics and are not necessarily related to respiratory disease (which includes conditions like asthma and COPD), but they can be.

Breathe with, not against,
an uncomfortable feeling.

Close your eyes and think of something in your life presently that causes you some anxiety or stress. Now notice your breath as you linger on that thought. Are you holding your breath in? Is it tight? Shallow? Heavy? Keep holding that thought and breathe with it, rather than trying to put the feeling out of your mind. Think of your breath as a companion to the feeling, right alongside it, even if doing so is painful or uncomfortable. Allow slow and comfortably long breaths as it stays with you, giving the feeling space. Stay here until there's a softening and your breath feels more open, less tight and restricted.

Natural Patterns of Breathing

We each learn distinct ways to adapt and manage our individual circumstances with our breath, but as humans, we also have universal breathing and nervous system responses. We all respond to the feelings and emotions listed below with similar patterns of breathing. Knowing this can be helpful for emotional regulation. Here's how the body is designed to breathe as it responds with the autonomic nervous system:

HAPPY: Breath is slow, easy, and full.

RELAXED: Breath is quiet, softly shallow, and slow in the abdominal area.

ANGRY, FRUSTRATED: Breath is fast, tight, forceful, and higher in the chest.

AFRAID: Inhale is fast or sharp; we hold back the exhale and keep it shallow.

STARTLED: Breath on the inhale is more like a gasp.

TENSE: Breath is shallow and tight on the inhale *and* exhale.

These ways of breathing are natural. This is what it means for our breath to be responsive, when we can easily move from emotion to emotion without getting stuck in one. Sighing and yawning are also signs that the body is naturally attempting to balance. Sighing is a form of exhale that kicks in when we need to let the air out; yawning opens the body and stretches the lungs to take a deeper inhale and activates the vagus nerve to feel more relaxed and alert.

HOW RESTRICTED
BREATH PATTERNS FORM

Each of us develops our own ways of meeting the need for safety and security—from the microcosm of our childhood experience of family to our adult sense of identity and belonging in the world. But the patterns of tension your breath, body, and mind hold were never originally in your control. Rather, these protection responses and habits grew from your instinctive attempt to attain a sense of well-being in your environment, whatever that environment was for you. For example, as we go through life, we have difficult experiences, and so we contract or tighten. Every time we contract, we hold our breath. Over time, we can develop habitual breath-holding patterns. Our body remembers our experiences, and our thoughts and beliefs can keep our restrictive breath patterns in place. Our stress-holding habits can become so familiar, we often don't realize that we are engaging them.

When we are consistently holding our breath, our posture is also affected. Our core breathing muscles make up most of our postural muscles—the abdominal, diaphragm, and pelvic floor muscles, and the muscles that run along the length of the spine from the neck to tailbone. Our ability to sense what's going on inside our bodies, physically and emotionally, or interoception (see page 39), can allow us to catch and release our stress patterns by responding in a self-supporting way.

One experience stands out in my mind whenever I think about how unaware we can be of our own patterns. Years ago, I taught a lunchtime breathwork class in a nursing home. I was teaching the residents to breathe from the diaphragm and to recognize how the abdomen moves outward with the inhale. As I walked around to assist people, I noticed an eighty-five-year-old woman who was breathing in the opposite way. When I pointed out her reverse breathing pattern, she said that it was the silliest thing she had ever heard. She insisted that she was breathing just fine. She couldn't feel that she was breathing in an inverted way, or understand what the difference was. She had a hard time feeling her posture or body at all, which demonstrated to me how breathing the opposite of the way we are designed to breathe can cause an extreme disconnection from the body.

Multiple factors impede free-flowing breath, ranging from the physical, such as muscle tension and injury; to specific respiratory conditions, including asthma, chronic bronchitis, and emphysema; to the emotional—chronic stress, fear, anxiety, guilt, anger, and unresolved trauma. Mentally, we restrict our breath via our thought patterns: critical self-talk, for example, generates tension, self-judgment, and defensiveness. On a spiritual level, we may hold our breath and tense our body when we feel disconnected from our deeper sense of meaning or being, inner peace, and loving presence, whether through nature or anything else we consider sacred.

No matter how tight and deep our breath patterns are, however, each of us can learn to repattern them. It's simply a matter of recognizing that these patterns are not entirely fixed. Rather, they developed over time because there was not awareness of them. The same inner intelligence that helped you survive remains alive and well within you in this moment, ready to be called upon to support new, unrestricted and open patterns.

REPATTERNING THE BREATH

Just as patterns of contraction develop from holding and breathing the same way over and over again, repatterning also results from repetition. By *consciously* opening the breath and freeing it repeatedly, a more consistent and open breath can become your new normal. When I work with a client, I look for where the breath is moving and where the flow of breath is blocked in the torso and throat. Typical breath patterns often reveal themselves after just a couple of minutes.

You can learn much about a person by observing their unconscious breathing patterns. I have seen how these patterns go hand in hand with belief patterns based on life experiences. I often witness the same breathing patterns in families, with parents, children, and siblings all adopting similar traits. In order to relax your own holding, start by observing your body and breathing with awareness, then be curious about the emotional connection. Restricted patterns will show up most often under stress or fear, for example, or when we're wracked with self-doubt or anxiety. Others are more subtle and chronic.

Identifying Restricted Breath Patterns

The more we revert to compromised breath patterns, the more these habits become regular tendencies. The following are some common restricted breathing patterns that I have observed. Read the description of each, and notice if you recognize any of the traits in yourself. Then act out each one to see whether it's familiar or comfortable to you, a constant habit, or something that manifests only once in a while. It may feel strange to purposefully try the posture and the breathing, but it helps you recognize your own patterns and have empathy for others who have different ones. In time, the more often you catch yourself and respond with a freer pattern, the less you will be able to tolerate the restricted breath.

Pay attention to your thoughts as you go through the exercise. Stay curious, and ask yourself how you feel. The "interrupt it" suggestions are meant as guidance and an orientation to repeat as often as you can in order to develop new ways of breathing. Consider consulting with a breathwork practitioner if you want to go deeper in exploring and opening your habits of breath holding.

Chest Breathing, or Holding Up

The inhale initiates and moves in the chest, and the abdomen remains tight.

BREATH PATTERN: This pattern presents as shallow chest breathing, as a result of tightness and tension holding up the abdomen and keeping the diaphragm tight and the lungs from accessing a full breath. Tension also lifts and holds up the shoulders, chest, and neck on the inhale, without much letting go on the exhale. The primary breathing muscles are bypassed by the smaller, secondary (or accessory) muscles, so the breath has to work harder and faster, utilizing only the upper portion of the lungs. The result is subtle or extreme overbreathing (hyperventilation), which pushes out too much carbon dioxide and offsets its balance with oxygen. There's a tendency to get caught in the stress cycle, which causes us to feel emotional distress, anxiety, and fatigue.

BODY HABIT: The posture is straight but tight, and the spine tends to be stiff or rigid. It can look like you're standing at attention with slightly lifted shoulders. There is sometimes slight tension in the front of the neck or throat when you're speaking or just breathing. It can be hard to calm down or stop the mind from worrying. Spinning thoughts may make it difficult to fall asleep at night. There can be a tendency to feel tired in the middle of the day.

TRY IT ON: Take a few breaths, inhaling and exhaling up into your chest without moving your abdomen. Notice how you feel. Now lift and tighten your shoulders about ¼ inch (6.5 millimeters) and try to relax your exhale all the way out. Hold that and try to inhale freely. Notice the area that moves when you inhale. Now take 5 breaths like this. Notice how you feel. Shake it off and breathe naturally.

INTERRUPT IT: Help your body remember to breathe slow, low, and easy, feeling expansion in the lower rib cage and a soft belly with the inhale. Give your shoulders to gravity. Relieve the upper-body tension by softening the chest ribs with the exhale. The practices in chapter 2, including Freeing the Exhale (page 72), Wake Up the Respiratory Diaphragm (page 86), Wake Up the Belly (page 88), and Wake Up the Pelvic Diaphragm (page 89), will help you to remember diaphragmatic breathing.

Rushed Breathing, or Holding Fast

Before the exhale finishes, the inhale rushes in.

BREATH PATTERN: This form of chest breathing is a perfect example of how the pattern directly reflects when we feel there's never enough time, because the exhale doesn't get to land into relaxation. With the nervous system in constant "go" mode, it's difficult to relax, settle into the body, and achieve a sense of balance. It can also feel as though there's not enough space for yourself in your life.

BODY HABIT: Since this is a form of chest breathing, the posture is similar, with tension in the upper body and shoulders. The body can lean forward slightly when you're walking, and there's a tendency to speak fast; both traits reflect being in the speedy sympathetic response. It's common to run out of breath when talking because the inhale jumps in before the exhale can carry the words out to the end of the sentence. It may be hard to focus on one thing for very long or slow down to be present in the moment.

TRY IT ON: Exhale, and when about half of the air in your lungs has emptied, immediately make your inhale come in. Repeat 5 times or until you start to notice the effects. Stop and notice what you feel in your body and mind. Shake it off and breathe naturally.

INTERRUPT IT: Focus on feeling the full completion of the exhale, giving it time to empty out all the air before the inhale flows in. Breathe with a balanced flow at an easy pace. Follow the practice Freeing the Exhale (page 72). Or try any of the practices that encourage a natural (not forced) inhale, like Wake Up the Respiratory Diaphragm (page 86) in chapter 2. Coherent Breathing (page 122) also helps balance your breath rhythm.

Collapsed Breathing, or Holding Down

The inhale is shallow and it's difficult to expand the breath out and up.

BREATH PATTERN: Breathing is generally shallow, especially on the inhale, as it's difficult to bring it up to get a full breath, which keeps the body's energy level low. When you're holding down the breath, inhaling fully can feel like too much work because the range of motion of the diaphragm is compromised. Any exertion at all can cause shortness of breath.

BODY HABIT: The upper body appears slumped to varying degrees, with the chest sunken in and the shoulders rolled forward. The breathing muscles and spine are pulled in and down in a way that inhibits full lung capacity and vital energy flow throughout the body. The diaphragm and core muscles tend to be weak. There can be a tendency for the abdomen to protrude and the hips to press forward. The spine is not supported by and does not hold up the body's frame. It may be hard to muster the energy for daily activities or to walk up stairs without running out of breath.

TRY IT ON: Standing or sitting, slouch and round your shoulders and sink your chest in, with your head a little forward. Now try to take a full inhale in this position. And then exhale. Notice how it's hard to expand the breath and more work to inhale. Repeat a few times until you notice the effects. It doesn't take long. Notice how you feel. Shake it off and breathe naturally.

INTERRUPT IT: Strengthen the flow of breath and open the posture. Focus on expanding the inhale and bringing your breath and energy up from the lower belly and into your body by opening your chest and lengthening your spine. Explore pressing your feet into the floor, then lengthening your spine (not shoulders) on the inhale. Let the exhale go while staying upright and open to the next inhale. Start with the practice Stretching to Make Space (page 92). Or use the movement practices in chapter 5 to open your body structure with breath, including Shaking (page 168) to energize muscles, and Rhythmic Walking and Breathing (page 175) at a brisk pace for more energy. From this chapter, Twist and Roll (page 118) is great for balancing the breath and postural muscles, and the Circle of Breath practice (page 126) is great for feeling vital energy flow and freeing the core muscles.

Contained Pattern, or Holding In

The inhale and exhale are so small that you barely see breath movement; the body is tight.

BREATH PATTERN: When I see this pattern, it appears like the breath is barely moving in the body. Contained breathing is marked by fast and shallow breath, pulling the life energy inward and holding it there. In extreme cases, this is known as a frozen breath and body pattern that can be an expression of a trauma response. Being outwardly expressive in the personality can be difficult or uncomfortable when your breathing (energy) is pulling you in the opposite direction (inward).

BODY HABIT: The posture is straight and pulled in, with shoulders and arms close to the body. The chest and whole outer body are held with tension. The body has learned through life experience that this way of holding is the safest way to be. There's a tendency to be more comfortable and connected in the mind than present in the physical body.

TRY IT ON: Hold your body as if you were standing outside in freezing weather without a coat on, or holding still in place after hearing an unexpected sound late at night when you're home alone. Feel your spine get rigid. Notice how your muscles and arms become still and squeeze inward. Pay attention to what your breath does. Stay still, without changing anything for a minute or two, and notice how you feel. Now keep your body tight like this and try to completely relax your breath for 3 breaths. Hold your breath shallow and small as you try to relax your body completely for 3 breaths. Imagine walking through your day holding and breathing in this way. Shake it off and breathe naturally. If it's familiar to you, be compassionate toward yourself, knowing that it's never too late to open to the extent you want to and feel safe to.

INTERRUPT IT: Start by feeling the solidness of the ground under your feet, then focus on finding the safe, easy movement of the breath anywhere in the body. Explore the Hum and a Hug (page 64) and Self-Compassion Breath (page 144) practices to connect with the body and gently open the breath. Practicing the Breath Ball (page 165) helps you feel the expansion of the breath in a simple way. Moving the spine and body in an easy flow can also be helpful in freeing the tension.

Reverse Breath Pattern, or Holding Back

The abdomen pulls inward on the inhale, causing the rib cage and chest to lift upward.

BREATH PATTERN: This unconscious pattern, also known as inverted breathing, is a more severe form of chest breathing, in that the abdomen is not only tight but actively pulls in and up on the in breath, the opposite of our natural way of breathing. Rather than expanding and opening with the inhale, the abdominal muscles pull in tight, which disrupts the organic movement and function of the diaphragm and internal organs. Over time, this can cause multiple health conditions, including digestive problems, organ dysfunction, and confused thinking because the brain is not getting the oxygen it requires. Reverse breathing may result from a respiratory condition, like emphysema, where the dysfunction causes the breathing muscles to make drastic efforts to take a breath.

BODY HABIT: As a response to the lifted contraction of the diaphragm, the spine is tight and the pelvis may be slightly tucked. The chest is also tight, as the shoulders pull forward with the muscle tension. Since the breathing muscles and overall movement of respiration are not in their natural coordination, the sense of coordination in the body can be more of a struggle, for example, when trying to learn a dance step or catch a ball. The body has to breathe faster as an attempt to get the oxygen it needs, keeping the nervous system geared toward the stress response. There can be a tendency to get disoriented easily or disconnected to body awareness.

TRY IT ON: Inhale and pull your abdomen inward and up and notice what happens with your rib cage and upper body all on their own. Exhale and make your abdomen move outward slightly. This movement doesn't have to be big. Notice how it feels, especially in your gut area. Repeat 5 to 10 times and notice how the flow of your breath feels. Stop, soften your belly, and breathe easy and feel what you feel.

INTERRUPT IT: Focus on expanding the belly outward on the inhale and relaxing it on the exhale. With your hands on your abdomen, say to yourself as you breathe: "Inhale outward, exhale inward." Repeat multiple times throughout the day. And explore the Wake Up the Respiratory Diaphragm (page 86) and Wake Up the Belly (page 88) practices to help your body remember the coordination of your breathing muscles. Be patient, taking gentle breaths to soften any forcing or pushing.

Optimal Posture for Breathing

The ideal posture to support optimal breathing is one that is soft and open and not compressed (collapsed breathing) or rigid (chest breathing). Sit comfortably and imagine your head is a helium balloon floating to the ceiling. Your spine is the string falling toward the ground. The center of your breathing is low in the abdomen and lower rib cage. Keep your chest and rib cage open and your elbows a bit away from your sides. Explore slightly moving your elbows outward as you inhale and inward as you exhale to help your body feel the space inside your ribs. With your shoulders, seat, and feet sinking into the ground, take a breath.

It's just as important to have a long, soft, fluid spine and neck while giving your shoulders to gravity and your body to the ground.

LOOSENING STRUCTURAL HOLDING PATTERNS

The following pair of exercises is designed to loosen the spine and breathing muscles and encourage whole-body breathing to make way for repatterning the breath. Lie on the floor or ground for each. With that solid support, the muscles that keep your body and breath contracted get the message that they can let go, that they don't have to constantly hold you up against gravity. Slowly moving the spine and rib cage in this way also helps release the diaphragm and open the breathing spaces.

PRACTICE
Tuck and Rock

In tandem with your breath, this movement loosens the breathing muscles, where the diaphragm attaches to your rib cage and spine and soothes your system, breaking down any rigidity you're holding from the tailbone to the neck. I practice this every morning before I get out of bed and later in the day while lying on the floor.

» Lie on your back with your knees bent, feet flat on a mat or comfortable surface on the floor and head in line with your spine. Take a moment to feel your breathing. Feel the places where your body is touching the floor, and give them to the ground.

» Gently tuck your pelvis under to feel your lower back press into the floor as you exhale. Release slightly and gently arch your lower back, rocking on your sacrum toward your tailbone as you inhale.

» Tuck under and exhale as your belly relaxes in, then rock toward your tailbone with a slight arch and inhale as your belly expands. Continue to tuck and rock as you breathe. Feel your breath and movement flow together. Feel the movement and massage through your spine all the way to the back of your head. Find an easy and comfortable rhythm, and continue for 3 to 10 minutes.

» Rest and keep breathing without the movement for a few breaths, expanding your belly as you inhale and softening it as you exhale. Then let it all go and notice your natural breathing. How do your body and breath feel different? Is there more ease?

PRACTICE
Twist and Roll

Here's another everyday exercise, one of my favorites, to loosen the spine, neck, abdomen, rib cage, pelvis, and attachments to the diaphragm and help your breath flow more easily. Noted breathing specialist Carl Stough (see page 66) used this technique with his patients and clients.

» Lie on your back with your knees bent and feet flat on the floor. Breathe through your nose. Notice how your breath feels: Is it tight or easy, deep or shallow?

» Clasp your arms straight over your chest. Twist your arms and head one way and your knees the other way, turning from your waist.

» Switch sides and continue the side-to-side twist in an easy, comfortable rhythm—not too slow, not too fast. Keep your jaw and body as soft as possible. You will know when it doesn't feel like effort. Inhale to one side and exhale to the other.

» After 5 to 10 breath cycles, change and inhale and exhale to opposite sides. If you get confused, just breathe in and out in a way that feels good. Repeat side to side for 10 to 20 breath cycles (or longer, if it feels good).

» Then hold the position to one side. Rest there and breathe into the side of your ribs that faces upward. Take 5 easy breaths into your ribs and torso. Take your time. Feel the movement as you breathe. Stretch to the other side and repeat.

» When you're done, rest, lie on your back, and breathe naturally. Notice if the breath and body feel different in any way.

Tracy turned to breathwork for help with the stress of her demanding job. Her usual coping strategy was to stay busy, taking care of everyone *but herself.* She was aware that she held her feelings in and had trouble identifying her needs. Growing up in a large family, Tracy was never the center of attention or activity. When she did get attention, she spoke in a soft, gentle voice, to not bother her mother, and she still speaks that way today. Her childhood experience left her with the belief that she was on her own, with no external support. When she was young, she had to draw herself tightly inward to feel safe.

During our breathwork session, she quickly went into the contained, frozen pattern. Her whole body clenched as she got very still; her breath was imperceptible. She pulled her breath inward, where it felt safe to conceal her feelings. Her intention for breathwork was to be able to express herself and her feelings clearly rather than freeze, shut down, and be numb to her needs.

Acknowledging her desire helped, but her breath remained very small and shallow. I suggested she wrap her arms around her rib cage, inviting her to feel the warmth of her arms and hands and then find any movement of her breath, however small or difficult that might be, within the hug. Even if she couldn't speak or move, the soft movement of her breath was there with her, and she said it felt good to feel. Finally, I asked her to notice how her breath and body felt when she heard a few phrases: "You deserve loving-kindness," I said. "Just as you are, all parts of you. Feel the truth in those words, in the midst of that deep place of silence. Feel the breath moving as it is within you." She softened and felt more energy as her breathing grew easier. We continued with a gentle, flowing, connected breath, letting it move out from the center of her belly through every part of her body. She said she felt more present in her body, much calmer, and more hopeful. I suggested she rely on the memory of this nurturing breath when she needed to feel support.

She continued to practice this on her own, and she's now more willing to ask for support at work and is exploring vocalizing her feelings to everyone in her life. The key to unfreezing Tracy's breath pattern was helping her access the safety of the essential energy that she had long held deep inside her body.

WAYS TO REPATTERN

Even though this whole book supports healthy breathing, the following practices are powerful ways to repattern. Coherent breathing (for relaxing and balancing) and conscious connected breathing (for freeing and actively unwinding) both—shared here as the Circle of Breath practice (page 126)—help to change and balance the rate and depth of your breathing.

PRACTICE

Coherent Breathing

Coherent breathing is a form of paced breathing, which includes any exercise where you take slow, even, deep breaths using simple counting. Coherent breathing has been used successfully for years to create an optimal state of energy and relaxation. It regulates the autonomic nervous system (ANS) by maintaining a balance between its two branches, the sympathetic nervous system (SNS) and parasympathetic nervous system (PNS). (It has also been successfully used to treat patients recovering from traumatic events.) The steady rhythm of 6 breaths per minute synchronizes the heart with the breath, the blood pressure with the heartbeat, and the brain waves with both. Coherent breathing also maximizes heart rate variability and any habits of breath holding begin to soften and release with regular practice. This internal synchronization has been traced back to many cultures and spiritual practices that use this same rhythm of breathing, including the deep meditation practiced by Zen Buddhist monks, chanting the Hail Mary and reciting the rosary in Catholicism, and numerous mantras in yoga.

The practice is very simple. To prepare, sit comfortably and allow your breath movement to gently find its way to your belly and your lower rib cage. Keep your chest soft. Invite your breath to flow slowly through all this space as you practice. Contact and rub the areas with your hands, if needed, to feel the breathing spaces. Then let your hands rest on your belly as you breathe in and out through your nose. The counting gives your mind something to focus on and keeps your breathing steady. (You can find music created for this practice; try searching for "2 Bells," by Coherence on Spotify or Apple Music.)

» Begin by breathing in for 3 slow counts (seconds), then breathe out for 3 counts. Repeat 3 times.

» Breathe in for 4 counts and out for 4 counts. Repeat 3 times.

» Increase to 5 counts per inhale and 5 counts per exhale. If this feels too difficult, stay with 4 counts and slowly build your way up to 5 counts.

» Stay with this for at least 5 minutes and work up to 20 minutes a day. Finish by breathing easily and naturally for a few moments. You can also practice this for 5 minutes 2 or 3 times a day.

Conscious Connected Breathing

The practice of conscious connected breathing involves inhaling and exhaling without any pause in between to expand breath and energy into contracted areas of the body and mind. It is a deep repatterning exercise used to relax, unwind, and interrupt restrictions and holding patterns, welcoming expansiveness and freedom in their place. These days, a variety of schools have evolved from and teach this breathing method, each with its own framework and names to describe it. Some methods incorporate bodywork, specific coaching, or other therapeutic practices. The conscious connected breath is often used for personal growth and self-exploration. The effects vary from shifting into an experience of deep self-awareness, relaxation, peace, joy, and vitality to expanded and altered states of consciousness when practiced at a faster rate. It can be used to bring balance and healing on physical, emotional, mental, and spiritual levels, and can contribute to the potency of every breath practice you engage in.

Conscious connected breathing is practiced with holding a positive intention, grounded in the perspective that each of us has the innate potential for healing. This is what it means to have the experience of wholeness.

» The inhale and exhale are connected, with a pause in between.

» The inhale is active and flows through all the breathing spaces with an easy expansion of the belly, rib cage, and chest.

» The exhale is a letting go and falls without effort. Think of a little waterfall.

» The breath flows in and out through the same opening, either the nose or mouth. Breathing in and out through the mouth creates a more open flow of breath, simply because it's a bigger opening; it can also address tension patterns in the jaw and throat.

The pace or rate of breathing will determine its effects. Traditionally, and in my experience, conscious connected breathing has used a fast-paced breath pattern that's referred to as "purposefully hyperventilating." There's more variation in the pace nowadays in different schools of breathwork. A faster breath rate will access more energy flow to stimulate the SNS response, which is used therapeutically to assist in releasing repressed energy and emotions and to explore altered states of consciousness. A slower pace will stimulate the PNS, or balance the PNS and SNS to open the body for relaxation and more energy while still having the ability to release deep tensions and emotions. To introduce this practice in a book, I feel it's important and responsible to encourage a gentle version with an easy flow. The goal is to cultivate a freer flow of breath so that you can experience the ease, spaciousness, relaxation, and impact of this process for just 10 minutes.

As your body opens to more energy and oxygen, you may feel sensations like buzzy, tingly, hot, cold, trembly, or waves of energy that feel good, or tension that your body wants to release. Breathing this way may bring up emotions or tears. Breathe with them, giving them space to be present. This energy knows how to move through you. Your body wants the freedom to let go of what it has been storing.

Let your breath welcome whatever thoughts or feelings arise during the practice. When thoughts come forward, they may be a distraction or offer an opinion about what you're doing. Thank your mind for its opinion, and give it this breath. Breathing with those responses will allow them to pass through. You can stop anytime and come back to an easy natural flow of breathing. You are in charge.

PRACTICE
Circle of Breath

This is a guided gentle version of conscious connected breathing. In this practice, keep your body relaxed as you breathe without pushing, forcing, or straining. This allows your breathing muscles to find one another and to work together to open your lung capacity and circulate oxygen and energy throughout your body. As energy moves inside, it can be normal to feel a little buzzy or light-headed. At any point if you feel overwhelmed or any discomfort, stop, breathe naturally through your nose, and rest, putting your hands on your body, belly, or chest and feeling the contact of the ground under you, supporting you, for a few minutes. Then move and stretch before getting up. It can take time to expand the body's capacity to open the flow of breath energy. If this practice is new to you and you want to explore a longer session, seek a breathwork facilitator to guide and support you in the process.

» Start by setting an intention: Ask yourself what you would love to receive or open to from this practice. More energy? More ease? Relaxation? Connection to yourself? Peace? See what comes to you after asking yourself this question. A willingness to open to whatever shows up can be enough.

» Create a pleasant, safe space for yourself, free from noise and other distractions. (The exception to this is putting on some music that you enjoy and that matches the pace of the practice or something that flows and feels good to you—for example, cello, violin, piano, anything with a light rhythm—and breathing with that. Be moved.)

» Lie on your back on a comfortable surface. If you need support for your lower back, put a pillow under your knees to relax your lower back or bend your knees with your feet flat on the floor. Feel the ground holding and supporting your whole body—every muscle, every bone, even your head. Move your jaw around and yawn if you can feel the open space in your throat, then let it soften and open.

» Begin to breathe in and out through your mouth in a gentle flow. For a sense of flow, start with an easy rhythm, inhaling for a count of 3 or 4 and letting the exhale fall out like a sigh of relief. Let your exhale land without holding it before the inhale. If you like, take more time.

» After a few cycles, your body will find its rhythm, and you can let go of the counting. Keeping the breath steady and connected is the key. Think of a big waterwheel with water flowing in, falling out, flowing in, falling out, as the breath flows through you.

» Imagine an open channel from your jaw and throat that's as wide as your rib cage and your hips. Breathe from the back of your throat only as deep as and at the rhythm that feels comfortable to you. Explore that for a few breaths.

» Now rub each area of your lower abdomen, lower rib cage (solar plexus), and chest with your hands. Rest your hands on each area; feel the warmth, and invite 3 breaths under your hands at each one. Inhale with a relaxed expansion, and soften as you exhale.

» Rest your hands and arms by your sides or wherever they are comfortable on your body. Continue to breathe in this gentle connected flow from your throat to your belly and through your rib cage, expanding like a balloon in all directions. Flowing in and expanding, falling out and softening back in. Let the waterwheel of breath flow through you as you become aware that you're receiving life support as you inhale. Allow the exhale to fall freely from the top of the inhale. From there, the inhale flows in from the bottom of the exhale like a gentle wave rising. Flowing in, falling out. Invite your diaphragm to be free. Notice what it does. At this moment you're nourishing your blood, your mind, all your nerves, all your organs, every cell, every part of you.

» Breathe in as much as it feels good. Breathe out; let it fall and cleanse your whole system. Breathe as deeply as feels good. You don't have to push beyond that, and you don't have to take in less than that, either. In and out. Nourishing and cleansing. How much feels good? Stay with that. What pace or rhythm feels good to you now? Follow that.

» Stay with this steady, easy flow of breathing for 3 to 10 minutes, then rest. Let the ground hold you. Let your breath flow naturally through your nose. Receive what's here for you. Take your time.

» When you're ready to move, begin to stretch, then slowly come into a sitting position. Once you're upright, notice how you feel different in your body than you did before the practice.

» Practice up to 10 minutes twice a week and work up to 5 to 10 minutes every day.

Therese had been diagnosed with breast cancer. After the shock of hearing the news, she had a deep desire to be able to accept the diagnosis. She decided to explore breathwork, hoping to open herself up to physical, emotional, and spiritual balance. In one session of lying down and breathing in a connected, steady flow, after she had just completed many consecutive days of radiation, she mentioned feeling vulnerable and uncomfortable during the treatment because her chest was exposed with male practitioners in the room. During this session, that deep sense of vulnerability began to surface. She instinctively put her hands on her abdomen and chest; the contact helped her feel the safety of her body's own boundary. As she kept breathing, her body began to shake, and she moved into deep crying, exhaling and releasing the emotions and deeply held tension in her body that she had been unaware of. As she stayed with the process, the waves passed and she relaxed into an easier flow of breath and a more peaceful state. At the end, she shared that this was the moment she knew she was safe. She felt more connected to herself with a sense of openness and joyful inner freedom. It was clear that she was now connected to the resilience of her innate life energy, free from the burden and contraction of the fear and emotions her body was holding.

A natural unrestricted breath is free to respond, open to adapt.

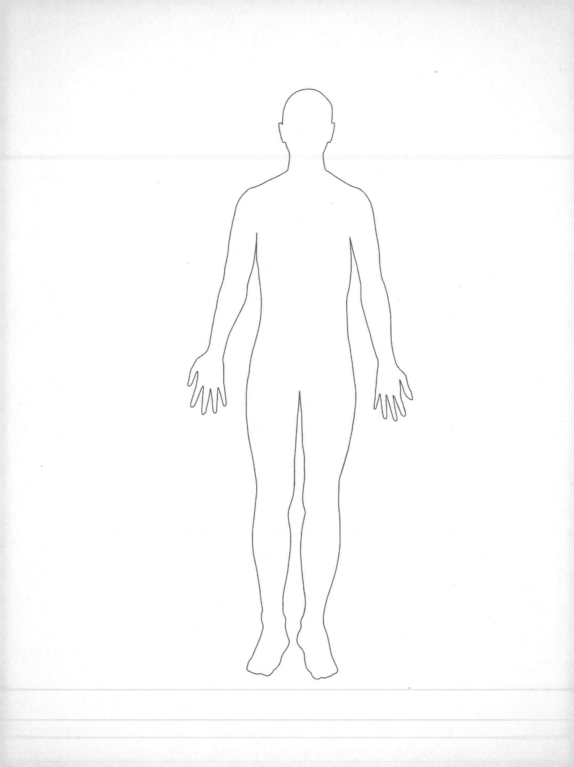

Your Breath

You have spent this part of the book waking up your awareness of your breath, discovering your relationship with it, and studying how it interacts with your body and nervous system. You learned to understand the influence of your unconscious breath patterns and habits of holding emotional and physical tension.

Use the body map opposite to see what you notice in exploring any of the awareness practices in part I. In my breathwork classes, I use this mapping exercise as a baseline check-in for students to assess where they are starting from. It's a powerful tool, because in order to fill in the map, you first have to feel into and connect to your breath and body in the present moment. Try it anytime you engage in a practice to track the quality, where you feel it, and sensations of your breath in your body before you begin, and record any changes you feel during or after.

1) Gently wrap your arms around your ribs and abdomen and feel the breath moving inside your body and arms.

2) Reflect on and respond to the following statements and questions by filling out the body map.

Using a pen, pencil, or any variety of colored marker, fill in spots on the body map to record what you notice about your breath in your body. To start, take note of where your breath is flowing and where it's not, giving you an overall snapshot of what your body is feeling right now. Where do you find your breath without trying to change it? Record if it feels tight, easy, deep, shallow, fast, or slow.

What breathing muscles can you feel moving now as you breathe that you weren't aware of before? What do you notice in your breathing spaces? Your abdomen? Intercostals (the muscles in between your ribs)? All through your rib cage and chest? Back? Pelvis? Are there spaces where you don't feel anything? Draw what you feel moving as you breathe.

In relation to your nervous system, show the places in your body where your breathing speeds up and tightens when you're stressed. Show where you feel your body calm down and soften as you slow your breathing and give more space to your exhale.

As you learned about breath patterns, what did you realize and feel into about your own breathing pattern(s) and how you habitually hold your body? Draw or color that in on the body chart or take a moment to journal about it.

Draw in anything else you became aware of about your breath within your body as you went through this section, like temperature shifts (warm, cold), range of thoughts as your breath changed, or something that surprised you that you didn't expect to think about or feel.

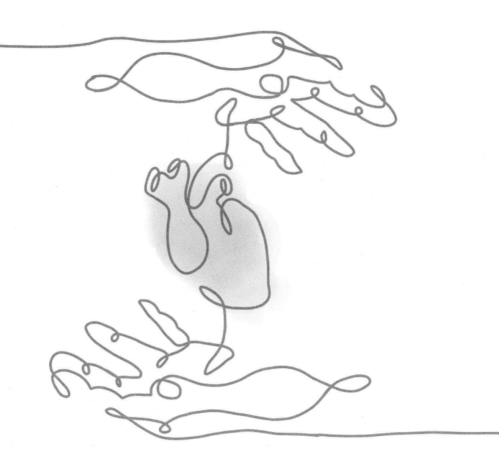

PART II

OPENING UP

Relax and be gentle. Breathe. Let your breath and heart rest naturally, as a center of compassion in the midst of the world.

—JACK KORNFIELD, *THE WISE HEART*

4

Being Kind to Yourself

Breathing as an Act of Self-Compassion

The foundation of my breathwork practice is the idea that giving yourself a conscious breath is an act of self-compassion, a way of opening up to meet yourself and those parts that you may want to push away. That's a kind response. This breath of love serves as a portal to the heart, through compassion for yourself and for others. The powerful combination of conscious breathing and self-compassion is at the root of self-care. When you combine conscious breath with a self-compassionate attitude, you have a skill you can rely on for the rest of your life. Your presence of mind when you breathe consciously will make a difference, and your motivation reinforces the effectiveness and experience of breathwork.

What's more, when the breath is open, we are more open to receiving self-compassion and knowing that we are taking it in as we breathe. By contrast, when we believe our own judgments and self-criticism, we are disconnected from our heart's access to acceptance and love and our body and breath tighten.

At some point as an adult, I realized that self-compassion was a much-needed, yet missing, link in my life. Throughout my childhood, there were unexpected emotional outbursts at home. I struggled so much in grade school that I often felt tight in my body with constant panic and anxiety. The physical effects of this stress hijacked my brain function and manifested as chronic knots and problems in my gut. My nervous system was stuck in the stress cycle (see page 55). This early experience with breathing and my own need for compassion led me to this path of practicing breath-work with self-compassion, now my life's work. Knowing that allows me to have deep compassion for my younger self and motivates me to help others who find themselves wanting to open their breath and places where they feel stuck. When we're ready, we can help those responses soften and relax.

Examining Self-Judgments

Feel your breath moving inside. Think of a familiar judgment or belief that you've held against yourself. What happens to your breath when you say it to yourself? Is there a place in your body where you can feel any tension from it? Now purposely invite your breath in to be with you as you touch these judgments. Notice what it's like inside your body to gently breathe, and stay with yourself in the midst of hearing harsh words. Keep breathing and notice if it's hard to stay with your breath when you believe this statement. That would be understandable, because we contract and hold our breath when we hear something hurtful. After a few minutes of steady breath, ask yourself if any of those statements are true. Keep breathing while you stay for a few minutes with the desire to know the truth about yourself beneath your beliefs about yourself. Write down anything you notice.

UNDERSTANDING
SELF-COMPASSION

The word *compassion* means "to suffer together." Compassion is the feeling of kindness and concern you would give to a friend who is struggling or in need. In those moments, an impulse in your heart moves you to want to ease another's pain. Think about how you show up for a good friend who is going through a very hard time. How do you talk to them? How attentive are you? What do you do with your body to show you care? Now think about how you show up for yourself. When you're in a difficult situation or feel as if you've fallen short of your own expectations, do you take a moment to try to ease your own pain? What do you say to yourself? How do you hold your body, your breath? Is there a difference between how you treat yourself and the way you approach your friend? The answer is most commonly yes. Why is it so difficult to give ourselves the same kindness, genuine concern, and reassurance that we offer to others?

Early in my practice, I found that bringing an attitude of compassion to the forefront was an important principle. In 2014, after years of exploring compassion-based practices, I began a formal study, enrolling in a program based on research by Dr. Kristin Neff, the author of *Self-Compassion: The Proven Power of Being Kind to Yourself* and a pioneer in the field. In 2003, Dr. Neff published a research article on self-compassion, the first of its kind. The findings offered a way to measure the benefits of self-compassion in a concrete way. Along with Dr. Christopher Germer, Dr. Neff created the 8-Week Mindful Self-Compassion (MSC) course, as well as an MSC teacher training program. After participating in the 8-week course, I was inspired to take the teacher training as well. Dr. Neff first defines compassion as being moved by another's pain, experiencing a feeling of kindness as our heart is connecting and responding to the urge to help in some way. That impulse turns on the motor cortex, the action part of the brain, which shows that compassion is not passive but an active response. We move toward the suffering of others with a desire to alleviate it. She explains that self-compassion involves the same qualities. It is the inner movement toward our own suffering, pain, and struggle for relief, a physiological response in the brain that moves us to act.

Anytime you breathe with rather than avoid painful and difficult feelings, you're turning attention toward yourself for support and relief, an act of self-compassion. Breathing with these feelings means staying in this uncomfortable place, rather than closing yourself off to it. Dr. Neff's research defines the three ingredients necessary for self-compassion. First is mindfulness, or awareness, to be able to recognize and acknowledge how we are feeling—that we are suffering. Next is common humanity, which is knowing that because we struggle, we are connected

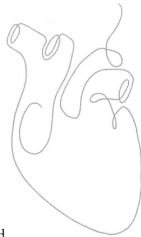

to all humans, that it's normal and we aren't alone. And finally, there's self-kindness, responding to ourselves as our own good friend giving ourselves support, care, and the comfort we need.

As I drew from this in breathwork sessions with clients, it became clear to me how the breath interplays with and reflects these three elements. Giving attention to the breath, and how it feels, helps us to develop mindful present moment awareness, allowing us to be more connected in our bodies and have the ability to better recognize feelings of pain and discomfort when they arise. Letting the breath meet those feelings to open, soothe, and nourish is a gesture of caring and compassion for ourselves.

Our breath is our most fundamental and unifying element—we share basic restrictions in breath patterns with each other. Being consciously connected with our breath will always be a reminder that we are not alone; that in this moment there are people (maybe millions) feeling and breathing in the same way we are.

Breathing with whatever you are feeling is an act of self-compassion.

Self-Compassion Breath

This practice is inspired by Dr. Neff's Mindful Self-Compassion program. It's a way to remember that you can give yourself love in the midst of experiencing any kind of pain or struggle, utilizing the breath and physical senses that comfort the body, with soothing touch and gentle voice. Gentle patting not only helps soothe and relieve tension but also helps you release trapped or stale air from your lungs on the exhale. This practice also helps to activate the relaxation response from the vagus nerve.

» Think of a situation that causes you to feel physical or emotional stress or discomfort. For the sake of trying it here, choose something that's not all-encompassing. It could be something connected to relationships, family, or work, for example. Or maybe it's an inner struggle, a self-criticism, or feeling like you don't have time to take care of your needs. This will vary for each person.

» Recognize it, be honest about how you're feeling, and notice if what you're telling yourself is causing more stress or tension. Notice the tone you speak to yourself in. Is it sharp, annoyed, edgy? Notice any sensations in your body. How does your breath respond?

» Sitting or lying down, place one hand on your chest and the other hand on your belly or the opposite side of your ribs, like a soft hug around your middle. Notice and feel the contact and warmth of your arms and hands.

» Begin to settle your body by gently tapping your chest with your hand in a soft, steady way, as if you were patting a baby's back.

» Inhale comfortably. As you exhale, make a quiet, comforting humming sound as your chest softens with each pat until the air is all the way out. Notice how the hum feels in your body.

» Let your next inhale come in naturally and feel that movement expanding gently inside your torso under your arms and hands from your belly, ribs, and chest. At the top of the next inhale, let it fall into the humming sound of the exhale down through your body like a warm, gentle waterfall as you pat. Feel the settling, the soothing, the safety. Repeat a few times until you feel an easy movement in your breath inside your body.

» Continue breathing in a slow, easy, steady flow, without humming, and say something kind to yourself, staying aware of the difficult situation you thought of at the start of this practice. Take your time and choose honest words that you can let in. Let your inhale help you receive the words. Let your exhale allow them to settle deeper. Say it again, then inhale and give it more space. If you can't think of anything to start, try, "May I be kind to myself in the midst of this."

» Keep speaking kindness to yourself, and exhale as your chest softens with each pat until the air is all the way out.

» As you breathe, practice remembering that whatever you are dealing with, you are not alone, because being in a place of inner struggle is something that you share with every person on the planet. And practice remembering that the ability to have compassion and give kindness is also part of being human. Breathe that in.

» It's okay if the judgmental part of you is trying to take over. Feel the hold of your arms and hands. Softly pat your chest and hum to it for 3 more breath cycles as you exhale. Gently let that critical voice be here, and know that you are still choosing to be kind to your whole self. Keep telling yourself the truth of your caring words as you breathe. Let them wash over you until you can begin to relax. Let your hands fall in your lap and your breath naturally flow with ease. Be settled. Be soothed.

THE REMEDY IS WITHIN US

Years ago, I took a forest foraging class in the foothills in Boulder, Colorado. As we were searching for edible plants, our guide explained that wherever you find poison ivy, you will find the antidote (he called it sticky weed) close by. I was amazed that nature would have the way to relieve discomfort and pain existing alongside its source. I forgot about this until I was sitting in a Mindful Self-Compassion teacher training course many years later and heard the instructor say that compassion is the antidote to suffering. Like distress and other challenges we may struggle with, suffering is part of being human, as are loving-kindness and the ability to have compassion for ourselves and others. The pain in your heart can be soothed by the same heart, where your compassion lives. The organic intelligence in our bodies orchestrates the remedy to the stress response through the relaxation response in the same location in the body—in the same area of the autonomic nervous system and our respiratory system. From this perspective, it's hard to argue that the natural wisdom of life is always with you, in you, and working for you. When we breathe with a benevolent intention, our inner wisdom and loving presence is given the space to do what it knows to do: open, calm, balance, heal, and revitalize us. In turn, the way we treat ourselves is reflected in how we treat others. Once we open with the breath, we are more open to receiving self-compassion. By contrast, when we believe our own judgments and self-criticism, we are disconnected from our heart's capacity for acceptance and love.

WHAT SOOTHES THE BODY

The power of soothing our own bodies is underestimated, so much so that for some, it might feel uncomfortable to consider it as a practice. Nevertheless, it's one of the most basic ways to begin to explore self-compassion.

Take the voice, for example: It can help us relax and settle or turn on the stress response, depending on the words and tone used. Research shows that comforting physical touch and a soothing voice incite the feeling of being cared for and release oxytocin, the "love hormone," whether for yourself or for someone else. This helps you shift out of SNS into PNS.

For some, it can take time to welcome touch if it's unfamiliar or associated with trauma. My mother never liked to be touched or massaged, but when she developed Alzheimer's, she forgot that aversion. When I rubbed her back, she would melt and say how good it felt and to keep going. I noticed that her breath slowed down as well. Without her usual defenses, her body remembered how much it naturally loved touch and could let go.

Consider this perspective: What if self-compassion is really about being willing to let everything you struggle with be held in love, not banished? Imagine all the love inside you, the kindest part of you, holding your most painful and darkest parts. Every part of us, including all the unloved parts, wants to come home to the light of our own heart, like moths to a flame. Sometimes when our heart opens after being closed for some time, our pain moves and comes up to the surface. It might feel disorienting or scary, or you may want to dismiss it immediately. That's okay—that response is more familiar than simply welcoming it in. This is when we hold our breath. But over time, your willingness to support yourself in this way and keep breathing will normalize a more accepting response. Keep in mind that we relax when we feel safe, and when we feel safe, we are okay with feeling as we do. Think of an upset child being held by a loving parent or adult who allows the feelings to be there, to simply flow through the body with the breath until the child calms down or "cries it out" and everything settles. This is the intelligent movement of our emotions when love holds them. As you understand how to use your breath to relax, balance, and open to your vital energy, your breath then becomes the warm welcomer to whatever inner experience shows up.

Being kind and compassionate toward ourselves softens and opens our breath and body.

Heart-Centered Breath

I practice this every morning before I get out of bed to feel grounded in my heart for the day. It provides a space for good intentions and space to be present, which helps remind you of what's important to you, and in turn will help you walk into each day ready to respond to others and to challenging situations in a more balanced way. By starting or ending your day with this practice, you're bringing your breath and intention into your center of wisdom—the heart.

» Sit or lie down in a comfortable position.

» Set your intention—in what way(s) do you want to open your heart today? Let your belly soften and take 3 gentle breaths, feeling the movement in your belly and lower ribs.

» Next, put your hands on the center of your chest/heart area and feel the contact and warmth.

» Inhale, taking a long, slow, and smooth breath, and imagine that it's working its way in from the bottom of your feet and the top of your head into your chest/heart area. You are pulling the breath energy up from your feet and down from the top of your head, the two flows reaching your heart at the same time.

» Exhale and feel your ribs soften downward under your hands, imagining and feeling your breath sink deeper and deeper into your heart. If it helps, you can inhale into your heart for 4 or 5 counts and exhale deeper into your heart for 4 or 5 counts.

» Repeat, and feel the breath flowing through your body in this way. Keep breathing into your heart area, allowing your breath to give space to your heart's intention.

» Stay with this for 5 to 15 minutes and notice any shift or feeling of centeredness, clarity, or ease.

VARIATIONS

Once you get the feel and flow of this practice, try adding intentional words or phrases for kindness, for heart intention, and to give a loving wish to yourself. Some of the following phrases are from Buddhist teachings, and others I have created in my own practice. Say them slowly as you breathe. You can inhale on a phrase and exhale on the same phrase, or try a different phrase for each:

May I be at peace.
May my heart remain open.
May I accept myself as I am.
May I remember that I am good.
May I be safe.
May I be happy.
May I be kind.

May I see what's true.
May I be grateful.

You can also inhale and exhale on one word like *peace* or *love*, or let other words of intention come to you. There might be no words, just the feeling of the breath flowing into your heart, or an image that appears instead of words. Just see what comes to you and welcome it in.

These phrases don't have to start with "May I be." Find and use meaningful words that feel good to you and that you would love to hear! Make this practice personal for what you need or want in the moment.

A BREATHWORK STORY

As the mother of two young boys, Beth struggled with her patience and feelings of guilt whenever she lost it with them. She hoped that working with the breath might calm her frazzled nerves and open up her shallow breathing. When we began our online sessions during the COVID-19 lockdown, she was downstairs in her home, while her husband and kids were upstairs. At one point, when she heard one of her boys screaming, she felt the impulse to run to him, even though her husband was there. It was upsetting to her that she couldn't let that go. I suggested she pause for a moment and notice where she felt she was holding on in her breath and body. Her breath was tight in her belly, and she felt tension in her chest and head. When I asked if she would be willing to give herself space for self-care, her shoulders dropped just at the thought of it. I guided her through the Self-Compassion Breath practice (page 144), which helped her soften and let go. Next, I guided her through the Circle of Breath practice (page 126). She reported feeling a fuller, freer breath. When we ended the session, Beth was excited to return to her family. In order to care for everyone else, she had to first learn to comfort herself when she needed to. Her perspective shifted when she moved her attention away from the outside and toward her breath and space within. She now relies on these practices regularly.

Imagine all the love inside you, the kindest part of you, holding your most painful and darkest parts. Let your breath open your space of love.

There is a vitality, a life force, an energy, a quickening that is translated through you into action, and because there is only one of you in all of time, this expression is unique. And if you block it, it will never exist through any other medium and it will be lost.

—MARTHA GRAHAM

5

Moving with the Breath

Shaking, Swinging, Walking, Tapping

When I was growing up, it seemed the only time I felt I was breathing freely was when I was moving my body. Playing sports and dancing were when I felt truly happy. Whenever I could move freely, I could breathe easy. Looking back, I realize that movement freed me from the flight part of my body's fight-or-flight response. The wisdom of my body showed me what I needed. Releasing my long-held breath fueled my body to keep moving, relax, and experience joy.

I followed that feeling through college and many years after, teaching fitness, disco (it was the late '70s!), aerobics (the '80s!), performing in a dance theater company, and studying yoga and qigong. Each pursuit added to the excitement of learning more about movement and breath, and I began to appreciate the dynamic combination of the two. This realization eventually set the course for my study of breathwork. During my very first session, I felt as I did whenever my body moved freely: open, happy, centered, empowered, peaceful, and connected to something bigger than my limited view of myself. I realized that my breath is at the core of this feeling of aliveness.

The truth is, this relationship is accessible to everyone, at every level of fitness and activity. Your breath is naturally stimulated by movement, and the way you breathe affects how you move. As we've learned, our respiratory muscles pump the air in and out of our lungs, as well as drive the body fluids like blood lymph. Our rib cage and breathing muscles are the house for our lungs, and we need to take care of that structure—opening it up and shaking out the dust, so to speak. The diaphragm is at the center, forming the core of the respiratory muscles and postural muscles. In order to function optimally, our breathing muscles need stretching and regular movement, just like every other muscle in the body, as well as the parts of our skeletal system that are connected to the diaphragm—namely, the spine, rib cage, and pelvis. Because our bodies become more rigid as we age, it's especially important to combine physical movement with conscious breathing to maintain healthy lung capacity.

What's more, the benefits you reap from exercise, including enhanced strength, endurance, and better muscle recovery, depend on the quality of your breathing—as do the ease and enjoyment you'll experience. Teaching aerobics classes taught me the importance of breathing in a steady, even rhythm; the same holds true for any aerobic activity, like running. With core strength-training exercises, exhaling on exertion creates stability for the spine with the core muscles, including your diaphragm. During activities like yoga, which involve moving and holding your body in different postures, taking long, slow, smooth breaths allows your muscles to stay soft and pliable as you attempt to stretch deeper and extend your range.

Building upon my own experience and training with movement-based practices, including qigong, yoga, and dance, I've adapted and developed the practices in this chapter. Though the steps and positions vary, the intent is the same: to open the breath and the body through movement, so that one supports the other.

As with all practices, listen to your body; if anything hurts or is uncomfortable, stop and come back to gentle, steady breathing. Modify to meet your level of comfort while giving yourself permission to explore stretching a bit out of your comfort zone, without straining. You can do one at a time or practice them in sequence. Experiment to see what feels best to you and follow that.

Many years of teaching movement classes have led me to understand how powerful it is when combined with breathwork practice. A few decades ago, I taught aerobic dance classes for stress reduction at an alcohol addiction treatment center in New York City. Twice a week as part of a twenty-eight-day inpatient program, I met with residents from a range of cultures and backgrounds who had very little in common. At the first class, everyone arrived quietly and kept largely to themselves. I began by putting on soft music, to accompany the warm-up of slow movement involving an inhale while lifting the arms and an exhale while lowering the arms. As the class progressed, the music did, too, leading into a variety of rhythms, with fast-paced drums and funky dance beats to encourage stretching, opening, and freely moving the body.

We formed a circle and kicked with "ha" breaths to help release tension and energy (see page 164). Halfway through the class, I invited volunteers to dance in the middle of the circle. As the weeks went on, one by one, everyone began jumping into the circle and cheering each other on. I knew that their breath was more open thanks to the freedom they felt to express themselves with the motivating music. It was so beautiful to see the shift as everyone mingled, talked, and laughed together, and I've long thought of this story as an inspiring example of our shared humanity.

Finding Your Rhythm

The pace at which you move through your daily life affects the rate of your breathing and your mental activity. We lose touch with our own inner rhythm when we try to keep up with the pace of life around us, or when we get lost in our thoughts, and disconnected from how our body feels. In order to find your own inner rhythm, you have to go inside your body to feel it. This helps you to catch yourself when you're disconnected from your natural pace as you move through your day. This three-part exploration is eye-opening for people in breathwork classes. When students walk around quickly or slowly, they most often look down at the floor as they try to match their idea of what that is. When they walk at their own rhythm, however, they have to feel, not think, and I notice them looking up and at each other more. They are more comfortable while moving in the more relaxed parasympathetic response, where connecting with others feels safe and nourishing. Finding your own steady rhythm of moving helps to balance your brain.

You can also replace these walking instructions with the intention of finding your own comfortable breathing rhythm. This exploration is helpful for practicing Circle of Breath (page 126).

» Find a space that's big enough to walk around in. Begin walking at a fast pace, then go a little faster for at least 30 seconds. Notice how that feels and bring your attention to any sensations in your muscles or elsewhere, to your breath, to your thoughts. Stop. Take note of what that was like and how you and your breath feel: Stressed? Comfortable? Uncomfortable? Normal?

» Next, walk around the room very slowly, then go a little slower for at least 30 seconds. Notice how that feels and bring your attention to any sensations in your muscles or elsewhere, to your breath, to your thoughts. Stop. Take note of what that was like and how you and your breath feel.

» Finally, walk around the room at your own pace. Give yourself a moment to find your rhythm. As you walk at that pace for at least 1 minute, notice how that feels, and bring your attention to any sensations in your muscles or elsewhere, to your breath, to your thoughts. Stop. Take note of how exploring that was different than finding a fast or slow rhythm—what that was like and how you and your breath feel.

OPENING THE BODY AND BREATH

The following practices are designed to open the body, increase energy flow, and boost your mood and mental clarity. Try any of them to start your day or as a midday pick-me-up. They can also help release tensions at the end of a long day. Keep in mind that they are meant to be nourishing and fun!

"Ha" Breath

This expands your breath and extends the exhale while also stretching your rib cage for more space as you inhale. It is a quick way to open your breath flow and clear your head. The breath is deeper than normal breathing; if you feel light-headed at all as you're breathing, start slowly and work your way up to more.

» Start by sitting with your feet flat, your knees open, and your hands palms-up on your knees. (You can also try this practice while standing with your feet open a little wider than hip-width apart and your knees slightly bent.)

» Inhale through your nose and lift your arms in front of you straight up over your head (or up to shoulder height, if you have shoulder problems) for 4 slow, easy counts, and exhale with a sigh sound, *haaaaa*, as you lower your hands down to your knees for 4 counts. Repeat 5 to 10 times.

» Rest, letting your hands relax in your lap. Breathe naturally. Notice any feelings in your hands or anywhere else in your body. You might sense some buzziness, warmth, or tingling—all are good signs that energy is moving.

VARIATION

» If you're fatigued or lethargic, try the following, which also helps release physical or mental tensions: Repeat the above practice at a faster pace. Breathe in fully through your nose while lifting your arms for 1 count (second). Breathe out through the mouth with a *ha!* sound while lowering your arms for 1 count (second). Start with 5 cycles, then stop and notice how you feel. Buzzy? Energized? Something else? If it feels good to you, do 5 to 10 or more. Then rest and feel what you feel. Let your breath come back to its natural flow. Stretch and yawn before you carry on.

Note: You can also lift your arms up and down, bending your elbows to your waist as you sit, stand, or walk around.

PRACTICE
Breath Ball

This basic standing (it works sitting or lying down as well) practice helps you feel the power of coordinated breath and movement using your hands. The movement of your hands helps to physicalize and allow you to see and feel the expansion of your breath and the rhythm of your breathing muscles moving in sync.

» Start by exploring with slow breaths at 4 counts in and 4 out, or at any slower rhythm that feels good to you. Breathe from the back of your throat with an open mouth and soft jaw, to create space.

» Begin by imagining there is a ball inside your torso. As you slowly inhale, the ball expands out in all directions: front, back, out to the sides, down, and up at the same time. As you freely exhale, the ball contracts back in place. The intercostal muscles between your ribs are stretching in all directions. Feel that for a few breaths.

» Now make a ball shape with your hands facing each other, close but without touching, fingers apart. Place them a few inches (about 7.5 centimeters) in front of your navel. Move your hands out slowly as you inhale into your belly, and move them in slowly where you started as your belly softens in with your exhale. Don't try to push the area open, but let your breath, body, and the movement of your hands be a slow and easy rhythm. Luxuriate in this breath with the movement for 5 slow breaths.

» Now move the ball in front of your solar plexus, expanding with your ribs out and in with your hands for 5 slow breaths.

» Move the ball in front of your chest, expanding out and in for 5 slow breaths.

» Then move it in front of your throat, out and in for 5 slow breaths.

» As your hands move in and out, bring your attention to them. Do you feel any sensations in your hands or anywhere else—buzzing, vibration, tingling? That's your life-force energy (qi).

» Relax your hands down. Imagine the ball expanding to fill inside your torso—front, back, sides, top, bottom—even if you can't fully feel it, stay with it; this will help your body begin to remember how you were born to breathe.

» Breathe naturally through your nose and notice if there's any sense or feeling of this synchronistic and coordinated rhythm of your breathing muscles moving together.

SHAKE AND SWING

The three practices that follow are inspired by my experience with qigong (see page 77). They combine movement, breath, meditation, and visualization to bring natural balance to the body, mind, and spirit.

PRACTICE
Shaking

Shaking is one of the easiest whole-body practices. The movement stimulates breathing, breaks up stagnant air or stuck energy in the lungs, rejuvenates cells, and energizes the body. Shaking will also oxygenate your entire body and can open you to your creativity. Use this as a formal practice as presented here, or more informally, like standing up from your desk or computer and shaking or bouncing your entire body, not thinking about anything but letting your breath flow and enjoying the movement in the moment. Even just 30 seconds can make a difference. People in my breathwork classes come alive with this practice. Playing high-energy music in the background (I love anything with percussion that's easy to bounce and shake to) makes the experience more fun and playful.

» Take a moment to notice how you are breathing now.

» Stand with your feet shoulder-width apart, feet flat on the floor. Start by lightly bouncing up and down on your heels (not slamming them down) while you shake out your hands in the same rhythm, like you're flicking water off your fingers. Make a *ha!* sound with each bounce. Repeat 5 times.

» Next, keeping your heels down, imagine you have little springs in every joint in your body—ankles, knees, hips, shoulders, elbows, wrists, fingers, jaw, base of the skull. Soften your knees and begin to gently bounce and shake your body. Your rhythm and movement should be comfortable and loose, not a tight shake. Your knees don't have to bend deep—just keep them springy.

» Keep shaking your whole body, allowing every part to be as loose as possible. Let your jaw and the base of your skull soften and gently shake out. Keep your neck soft and relaxed. Breathe easily from your diaphragm. Every now and then, while you shake and whenever your body wants it, open your jaw and throat and let out a big exhale, *ahhhhh*.

» As you shake and bounce, bring your attention and a few moments to focus on each of these different parts of your body:

- Imagine gently shaking and bouncing your joints free.
- Shake your muscles loose, releasing downward to the ground as you give in to gravity.
- Bounce and shake your bones and rib cage free.
- Shake your organs free of tension and give them space.

- Keep shaking and bouncing your whole body. Have fun with it. *Ahhhhh.*

- Practice for 1 to 5 minutes. Then stop and rest and feel the aliveness—the energy, buzzing, tingling in your body! Notice your breath. What did the shaking give you, and how do you feel different?

Swinging Arms

Swinging your arms loosens the tissue around the lungs and the muscles in the shoulders, back, and rib cage and opens the flow of circulation throughout the body. It can energize you or relax stress, depending on what you need. Rhythmic swinging is also excellent for mental clarity. According to Dr. Bessel van der Kolk, rhythmic movement helps to regulate our nervous system by shifting us out of fight-or-flight mode. This accounts for the brain's executive functioning, where we can think rationally, pay attention, make decisions, regulate emotions, solve problems, and take action.

Known as Ping Shuai Gong ("arm-swinging exercise"), created by Taiwanese qigong master Li Feng-shan, this simple exercise improves body circulation and boosts the immune system. The steady movement and breath together can center your mind and energy level.

Try this practice twice a day for up to 5 minutes at a time. Letting go of any muscular control of your arms and shoulders with the exhale facilitates letting go in general—of difficult emotions, stressful stories in your head, and the like. (Note: If you're new to the practice, you might feel light-headed; stop if that happens, even if it's after 30 seconds or a minute. Return to natural breathing. Otherwise, slowly build up to 5 minutes, or longer, if that feels good.)

» Stand with your feet flat and about shoulder-width apart. Keep your knees soft and springy. Breathe in and out through your nose.

» Inhale and bring your arms straight out in front and up to your shoulders. Think of your inhale energy (or qi) lifting your arms up.

» Exhale and let your arms fall and swing down without pushing or forcing. Let the weight of your arms and exhale fall with gravity.

» Continue with a fast but comfortable swinging rhythm (about 1 second per up and down), inhale arms up, exhale arms swing down. Keep your knees soft, lightly bouncing, as you swing.

» After every 5 swings, bend your knees slightly as your arms swing down and then bounce them gently back up as your arms swing up. As you stay with this, the swing starts to take over and can feel very energizing.

» Finish by coming back to a natural, easy breath, allowing your belly to be soft, with your feet supported by the ground. How do you feel different? How does your breath feel now?

Swinging Twists

This practice helps to loosen your spine, neck, and ribs, as well as the muscles in your torso, enabling your diaphragm to move freely and your lungs to fill easily. Twisting movements help promote healthy lymphatic flow.

» Stand with your feet shoulder-width apart, breathing comfortably through the nose. Start with smaller movements. As your muscles loosen, let your body open to freer, wider movement.

» Swing your arms from side to side as you twist freely, letting them fly open from your shoulders like scarves flowing in the wind. As you swing, move your head toward the twist and let one arm bounce off your back as the other arm bounces off the upper chest and shoulder. Repeat 10 to 30 times with a gentle flowing movement.

» Come back to stillness and allow your breath to flow naturally and easily. Rest and enjoy what you feel.

VARIATION

» Swing your arms freely up over your head with relaxed elbows as you inhale and down back behind you as you exhale 5 to 10 times. Then swing your arms any way that feels good—open front to back, diagonally, one arm up and down at a time. Inhale with the movement one way and exhale as you go the other way. Allow your spine and ribs to move freely.

Whenever you're moving and breathing consciously, something good is happening!

Gary is a veteran long-distance thru-hiker who was awarded the Triple Crown of Hiking for walking 8,000 miles on the three major US long-distance hiking trails. He came to me after developing reflux problems, which made it hard for him to breathe freely, especially while hiking uphill with heavy exertion. Hiking was a way to help calm his anxious thinking, but there were times when he would still get caught in the habit of worry and leave the enjoyment of the present moment. I taught him some breath and movement practices, including bouncing his knees and shaking (see page 168) to help his body let go. I worked with him to gently extend and release the exhale, and to inhale into and inside his belly and rib cage to find space for his diaphragm to breathe with the rhythm of his walking. His experience of emptying the lungs to allow more breath to come in helped him to keep his energy level even, which is especially beneficial during a 12-hour-long, 20-plus-mile hike. Afterward, he said that breathing fully while feeling his rib cage expand and contract with the rhythm of his hiking became a meditation. He also reported that his new way of breathing while hiking relieved his reflux symptoms effectively and gave him a sustained level of energy.

Rhythmic Walking and Breathing

Walking is one of the most common and beneficial ways to cope with daily stresses and uncertainties. Next time you're out for a walk, play with your breath. Let your body walk with the rhythm that feels good, which will allow your nervous system to regulate fairly quickly.

» Breathe through your nose, and let your arms swing freely by your sides, feeling the pull of gravity from your shoulders down your arms. Feel the easy movement in your rib cage as you walk. Let your neck be free.

» Find a pace that matches your energy level—high, low, or somewhere in the middle. For example, if you're upset or angry, try walking at a faster pace, 3 steps with the inhale, 3 steps with the exhale. Let your body move with that energy. Eventually your pace will slow as your nervous system regulates.

» If your thoughts are becoming a distraction, redirect your attention to synchronize your breathing and steps. As you walk, count how many steps feel good to you on your inhale and how many steps on the exhale—4 steps with a 4-count breath, for example. It doesn't matter whether your pace is slow or fast; just keep coming back to your body with an intention of walking with breathing to carry you, to support yourself.

Breath Dance

Explore this fun unstructured experiment anytime you want to feel inspired, stimulate your creativity, stretch outside your "box" of limited thinking, or simply breathe better.

» Start by sitting and noticing how your breathing feels: easy, tight, shallow, deep? Notice your mood and state of mind: happy, sad, open, closed?

» Put on a piece of music you love, rhythmic or flowing, that makes you want to move. Stand (or sit) still and begin to listen to the music—first with your ears, and then with your breathing as you notice how it changes and begins to dance inside you as you listen. Notice how the pace and depth of your breathing changes with the music. Follow your breathing and let it begin to move your body. You don't have to know how. Just

see what happens and go with it. Your body knows.

» Feel where the impulse to move your body arises: In your hands? Feet? Head? Arms? Torso? Take note of that impulse and let your body follow your breath. Or maybe your breath follows your body. Move to the music in any way that feels good to you. Move your ribs, your spine, your arms, your hips, anything, everything. Be moved! Be breathed!

» Keep moving until the song is over. Now sit and just notice your breathing and your mood. How is it different?

VARIATION

To open deeper, try this:

» When the music stops, sit or lie down, and begin to breathe in a gentle connected flow through your mouth, with a soft open jaw and throat as in the Circle of Breath practice (page 126). (You can breathe in and out through your nose, if that's easier for you.)

» As you feel energy in your body from the movement, let your breath flow in and flow out, expanding from your lower to upper torso.

» Continue breathing this way, receiving as you inhale and allowing your body to soften as you exhale, for 5 to 10 minutes.

» Rest for a few moments and breathe naturally through your nose; enjoy the flow of universal life energy in you now.

» Stretch your body before you get up. Write down anything you're inspired to record about your experience.

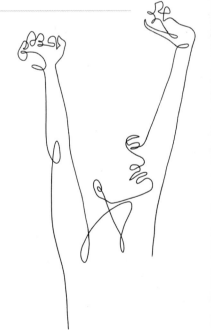

WHOLE BODY TAPPING

In qigong, tapping practice uses the fingertips, open-hand pats or slaps (with a loose, open hand), and soft fists in rhythmic percussion to stimulate and move energy flow. When you tap through a road-map-like system of acupressure points known as the meridian pathways, that energy is distributed throughout the body and helps to release tension and stimulate the skin, nerves, and muscles. In Swedish massage, a similar practice known as tapotement uses tapping, slapping, and cupping the hands to awaken the nervous system, break up tension, and stimulate the lymphatic system, the part of the immune system that protects us from disease and helps eliminate cellular waste.

All these methods help open and clear the lungs. Tapping the rib cage and lungs helps to break up and release accumulated carbon dioxide and mucus.

Use the following practices when you feel sluggish, distracted, or disconnected from your body; when you're experiencing brain fog or muscle tension; or anytime you need to wake up, focus, and reenergize. Truthfully, you may choose to do them simply because they just feel so good. Be sure to tap or pat gently but firmly—just enough to feel it penetrate your skin and into your tissue, not too soft or hard.

Tap and Pat

This practice is beneficial for waking up the energy flow and stimulating circulation in your whole body. The following steps are for standing, but you can also do this while sitting. (I find it keeps the breath flowing if you hum and then inhale when you need to as you tap and go through this practice.)

» Stand with your feet shoulder-width apart, with your knees slightly bent. Stay bouncy on your knees. (If sitting, keep your knees bent and your feet hip-width apart.)

» Start by rubbing your hands together, feeling the warmth in your palms. Now bring your open soft hands to your belly and, with loose wrists and relaxed shoulders, begin tapping, or patting, with open hands at an easy, comfortable rhythm on your abdomen 10 to 30 times to stimulate your organs. Try saying "one thousand one," tapping on each "one," to get to 2 taps per second.

» Breathe comfortably as you continue to tap and hum when you exhale to keep the breath flowing and inhale naturally.

» Place your left hand out in front of you, palm up. Tap your left shoulder with your right hand about 10 times and then tap down the inside of your arm to your hand (use approximately 10 taps to get from shoulder to hand).

» Turn your palm down and tap the back of your hand up the back of the arm to your shoulder. Turn your thumb up and tap down that side to your thumb. Bend your elbow and tap the outside of your hand on your pinky down to your elbow and then to your armpit. Tap your armpit about 10 times (this is good for your lymphatic system). Tap down and back up that side of your rib cage.

» Place your right arm out in front of you, palm up. Repeat the same steps as above on this side, down the inside of the arm, up the outside, down the thumb side, and down the pinky side to armpit.

» Cross your arms at your wrists, with loose fists. Tap your upper chest under your collarbones on each side, making a long *zzzzz* sound (like a buzzing bee) out loud until the air is all the way out.

» Next, inhale and lift your elbows, keeping your fists on your chest. Lower your elbows, tap with sound, and repeat 3 more times. The last time, make an *ah* sound out loud as you exhale.

» Relax your hands and tap both sides of your lower ribs.

» Tap your lower back area and down the back and sides of your legs to your ankles and feet.

» Tap up the front of your legs and inside your legs to your hips.

» Tap all around your hips.

» End with your hands on your belly. Rub your hands in a circle up the right and down the left a few times. Hold still here, feeling the warmth of your hands and softening your belly.

» Notice how your breathing feels in your body. Rest for a moment and feel what you feel. Enjoy the energy you just gave yourself!

» For brain fog, headaches, and overthinking, while humming, use your fingers and lightly tap all over your head—back, top, sides, forehead, temples, cheekbones, and jaw. Rest your hands on your head as you imagine gently breathing into your head for a minute. Relax your hands down into your lap, breathe naturally, and feel the effects.

Tension Tamers

These mini practices can be followed anytime you have just 30 seconds or a couple of minutes, not enough time to go through the sequence of a full practice. First, tap or pat the areas where you feel your breathing is restricted or any other place of tension in your body, such as your knees, chest, ribs, shoulders (one at a time), lower back, or hips. Next, make *ah* sounds or hum on the exhale. Inhale naturally and easily. Combine tapping your chest under your collarbones on each side (crossed wrists, soft fists) with light shaking or bouncing, knees soft. Tap points as you exhale (*ah* or *zzzzz* sound) and lift your elbows when you inhale. Try this 3 to 6 times.

Our rib cage and breathing muscles are the house of our lungs. Taking care of your house means opening it up regularly.

Heart Wings

This practice is designed to open your breath, stretch your chest and upper ribs, and loosen the muscles in the shoulders and upper back and the tissues around the lungs. It is also a good way to stretch your heart space open, physically and emotionally. When you need courage to take a big step forward in your life, try this practice as you hold that intention.

» Inhale through your nose while swinging your arms out to the sides and back, feeling the expansion of the chest as you lift your chin up slightly to open your throat.

» Stretch your fingers backward to open the energy pathways in the arms.

» Exhale through your mouth with a soft *ha* sound while swinging your arms forward and wrapping them around your chest. Let your hands bounce off your back ribs or arms as you slightly round your back and drop your chin and bend your knees a little more.

» Inhale as you swing your arms open and back again, lifting your chin slightly to open up your chest and throat.

» Continue flapping your arms open and rounding forward. When you find a comfortable rhythm, repeat 5 to 10 times, then come

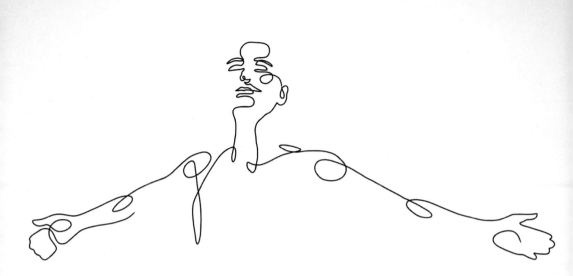

into stillness while holding your hands open in front of your chest, holding your heart's intention for a moment.

» Feel your feet on the ground, let your belly be soft, and let your breath flow naturally. Notice how you feel. What do you notice about your breathing? Enjoy this good energy in from your heart flow through your chest and body.

Your Opening-Up Chart

In part II, we looked at how conscious breathing naturally offers you the gift of opening, not only your respiratory system but your heart too, as an act of self-compassion. This intention gives you the space to let love hold every part of you, especially those you find hard to face or painful. We also learned the life-giving energy of moving and breathing in synchronized rhythm.

Opening up is a constant invitation for the expansive potential of your breath to connect with your heart and body, with yourself, to remember your shared connection with all life. Movement and breath are a loving way to give your body the joyful experience of aliveness in any moment. Use this diagram as a symbol of that invitation. Saying "I am open to breathe with . . ." is a way of affirming that you are here now, choosing to keep opening to the moment. As you think it and write it, become aware of where you feel and want to feel more openness to it in your body and in your life, and give it more open space with your breath.

1) Put your hand on your heart and gently breathe in an even flow, inhaling and exhaling, as you look at the openness wheel.

2) Reflect on and answer the following questions, starting each response by writing along the lines coming out from the center of the circle, where it says "I am open to breathe with . . ."

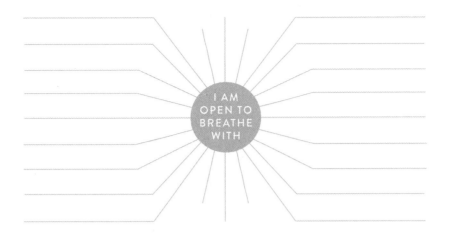

I AM
OPEN TO
BREATHE
WITH

State the ways and practice(s) you are open to doing in order to give yourself more compassion, more kindness with the support of your breath, for example, pausing in your day to do the Self-Compassion Breath (page 144) and Heart-Centered Breath (page 151) practices, giving yourself space and time to breathe while saying something kind to yourself when you are tightening against your self-judgments or fears, or rubbing your arms, belly, chest, or anyplace that feels soothing and comforting to you.

Of the difficult things you deal with, such as a persistent or worrying thought, an emotion like anger or fear, or a chronic physical discomfort or breath holding, which are you willing to stay present to and breathe with, giving yourself the message that "you" are here with you no matter what the discomfort? That willingness is your loving presence. What are you open to allowing love to hold anytime it arises within you? What practices feel supportive that you want to bring into your life?

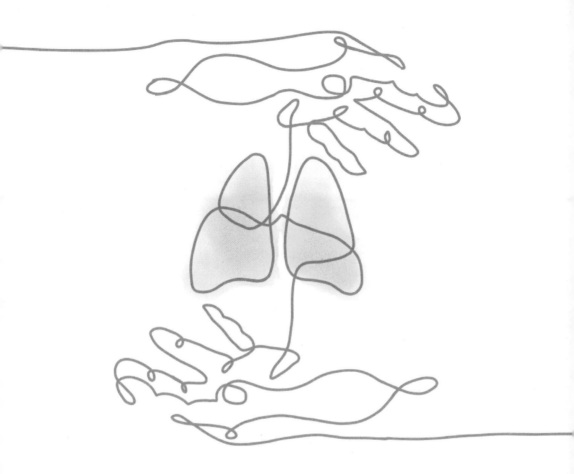

PART III

BRINGING THE BREATH TO LIFE

Breath remains the vehicle
to unite body and mind and
to open the gate to wisdom.

—THICH NHAT HANH

6

Relying On the Breath

Lifelong Tools to Carry You

Among the many benefits of breathwork is its portability. It goes wherever you go. Once you're aware of the power of breath, you can call upon it whenever you need it, anyplace, anytime, even just for a moment or two—no equipment required. Whether you're having trouble sleeping, anxious about events in the news, or stuck in traffic and late for an appointment, you can lean on your breath to move out of a state of worry and into one of relaxation. The unending support of the breath comes in handy whenever you need to slow down, get centered, and reset.

You may be familiar with the concept of a coping kit (or box), a collection of physical items to soothe heightened nerves or anxiety—close your eyes and imagine a soft blanket, scented lotions, a candle, maybe a pair of warm slippers. The breath works beautifully as a distinct kind of coping kit, one that exists right inside you. Just the security of knowing that this reliable companion is there for you can be reassuring and grounding.

BRINGING BREATH WITH YOU

As you carry it with you, the companionship of the breath helps you find your way back to the present. When you can come back into the present moment and connect with yourself, you're equipped to face life's challenges rather than feel defeated by them. You are more responsive than reactive, open to a more positive perspective, and able to choose kindness over judgment.

A breathwork routine practiced at a specific time can also make a big difference in how you feel. (For more on building a routine, see chapter 8.) A periodic formal practice will cultivate your mini moments of practice as you go through your day. I remind people of this all the time. Occasionally, a client will begin a session by admitting that they haven't practiced their breathwork since our previous session. In response, I ask, "Well, have you been aware of the breath more often since you were here last?" When they say yes, they started breathing consciously whenever they caught their breath tightening, I happily reply, "Well, that's it! That was your practice!"

DAILY BREATH BREAKS

At the Plum Village monastery in southwest France, cofounded in the early 1980s by Buddhist monk Thich Nhat Hanh, and the eight other Plum Village locations worldwide, the art of mindful living is taught and practiced. Mindful living is often referred to as the practice of awareness in the present moment. At Plum Village, at various times during the day, a bell sounds throughout the monastery, and everyone in the village stops and becomes aware of their breath. The purpose of this practice is to get your attention and to call you back home to yourself. By pausing, becoming quiet, and focusing on the physical sensations of your breathing and body, you can return to the present moment, wherever you are. When you take a moment to pause and find your breath, you give yourself space to find a calmer state of mind.

To adopt this practice, you might use a gentle bell tone on your phone, set to ring a few times throughout the day, or get an app for a bell to ring every now and then (Plum Village has a free app with this feature). You can also designate specific moments—when you wake up, at mealtimes, or when you're getting ready for bed—as reminders to pause and return awareness to the breath in the here and now, in order to feel peace.

We encounter unpredictable stressors all the time. In these situations, we're usually not present but instead find ourselves in a feedback loop of anxiety, worried about what might happen or triggered by past experiences. It is possible, however, to benefit from this state of mind—a judgment or a pain, ache, or tension in your body can serve as your bell sound, to bring you back to your breath and end the stress feedback loop in your brain and in this case, to remember kindness with the breath.

Breath Pause

To create your own moments of pause, follow and feel the full movement of the inhale all the way into the lungs and the full movement of the exhale all the way out of the lungs. Stay with it for 3 breaths, bringing attention to the present with each. Saying a few words might help you. Try any of these options:

» From Thich Nhat Hanh: "Breathing in, I know I am breathing in. Breathing out, I know I am breathing out." Or "Breathing in, I am aware of my whole body. Breathing out, I am aware of my whole body."

» Say to yourself as you inhale, "I feel my breath moving in my [area of body]," and as you exhale, "I feel my breath moving in [place within body]."

» Use one word for the inhale and one for the exhale, like "in-out," "open-calm," or "deep-slow."

» Find your own words—anything that helps you notice what's here right now with each breath.

COPING WITH INTERNAL FORCES

The more you begin to incorporate conscious breathing into your life in ways that work for you, the easier it will be to access and give your breath space to move more freely, no matter the circumstance. One breath response does not fit all, however. Follow and trust whatever

Pause,
catch yourself,
and
turn to
your breath as
an ally.

feels best as your breath becomes a more consistent ally. Sometimes, just softening your belly when you feel it tightening can help you breathe lower with more ease.

When you find yourself seized with an emotion or reaction, start with the following steps:

1) Pause when you catch yourself.

2) Acknowledge how and where your body and breath are reacting.

3) Notice what, if anything, you are telling yourself that's creating more tension.

4) Turn to your breath as an ally and give yourself a kind response.

Regulating Emotions with the Breath

The coping guidance here is specific to each situation, but it is based on the practices and information in the book. To start to use your breath as a coping kit, explore how it can help regulate difficult emotions. Read through the following list of emotional and mental states, along with the suggested responses to each, and practice the ones that resonate with you. As you explore each entry, become aware of common scenarios in your life that trigger each feeling. Curiosity about your own reactions and responses to these emotions creates the space for change.

Anger

Anger comes on fast. The feeling presents itself in your body as a rush of energy (adrenaline) that increases your breathing and heart rate. What you're telling yourself about the situation could be fueling it. The key is to help your breath become slower and more even.

- Notice the fast pace of your breath and consciously breathe with it a few times rather than trying to hold or push against it. It's like if you jumped on a runaway horse before taking the reins.

- If you can, move, stretch, or shake your body (see page 168) out as you breathe to allow the anger energy to naturally move.

- To help you slow down and unwind, start with your next exhale, focusing on extending it with a long *ah* sound, easy like a sigh rather than pushing it out. Let it flow out slow and steady. Soften your belly as best you can and inhale slow and long. If you're with other people, make a low, even whisper sound from your throat, breathing through your nose.

- Use paced breathing to steady your breath and nervous system by counting with your breath (see Coherent Breathing, page 122).

- Follow your breath, rather than any thoughts or reminders of the cause of your anger. Tell yourself you can come back and problem solve after you simmer down.

Fear

Fear is important to our survival, but sometimes it can take control. Fear is usually accompanied by thoughts of what might happen in the immediate or long-term future. You may get overwhelmed or feel unable to think or act. When you're afraid, the rhythm of your breath is interrupted by holding the inhale in and not releasing the exhale. First, bring your attention to the present—is the threat real or not? Body tension and swirling thoughts often make it hard to tell. Using your breath can help you connect to the rational, clear-thinking part of the brain, and tend to the feeling. Try the following to help your body turn on the relaxation response:

- Feel the ground under you and any solid support that's in contact with your body.

- Put your hands on your abdomen to help ground you in the present. Rub your belly in a circle if that feels good to you.

- Put one hand on your chest and softly lengthen the exhale through rounded lips (see Wind Tunnel, page 74) or a soft humming sound. Count the seconds on your inhale, and double that on your exhale. Slow, low, and steady. Soften your shoulders, jaw, and chest downward. That kind of letting go sends a message to your nervous system that you are safe.

- Wait for the inhale, and slowly guide it to move into your abdomen.

- Repeat a few times until you can find a quiet comfort at the bottom of the exhale and a fuller inhale. Even though the issue doesn't change, you are resetting your stress response to know you are safe right here and now. Your body and brain will be available to move forward from a more centered place.

Worry or Anxiety

When your mind is in panic mode and spinning out of control, your thoughts start to race and your body gets tight all over. This heightened state may be related to something specific in your personal or professional life or it might be general anxiety about what's going on in the world. Slow down and give yourself space by accessing the breath in the belly and lengthening the exhale. Start here:

- Rub your belly, chest, arms, and legs.

- Bring all your attention to feeling your breath moving inside your body, to be present. As you exhale, give your shoulders to gravity—just let them drop. Soften the muscles around your eyes. Imagine inhaling gently down toward your pelvic floor (as if a ball were expanding inside your abdomen, back, and pelvis).

- Give yourself space inside and practice whispering *la la la la la* at an easy slow pace as you exhale all the way out and soften your chest. When you feel the impulse to inhale, take it in low and slow into and out to the sides of your ribs without pulling it up. Let it then fall into the *la la la la la*s and repeat Freeing the Exhale (page 72) for about 10 breath cycles to help your body remember how to let go of the exhale with ease. Then rest.

Sadness

It's easy to forget that sadness, like all emotions, is something you share with everyone on the planet. Remember that you are not alone. When you're feeling sad, it's common to have difficulty breathing in or taking deep breaths. The effect is low energy levels and mood. Try to stay present and allow the feeling to naturally move through you as you create more space in your body with your breath. Letting yourself softly breathe with the sadness helps you relax with and accept what you're feeling. You are supporting yourself rather than getting over-taken by the sad thoughts, and your energy gets renewed.

- As you go through moments of feeling down, find your breath and breathe through your nose in an easy, steady rhythm of inhale and exhale, one breath flowing into the next, slowly and gently expand-ing your belly and ribs. Feel what you feel, noticing your thoughts and your body breathing at the same time. Do this at least 5 times in a row, or as many times throughout the day as you need for support.

- Use the Self-Compassion Breath practice (page 144) to give your body and the emotion support.

- Try the "Ha" Breath practice (page 164). Repeat 5 times, working your way up to 3 times a day to lift your energy and mindset.

Grief

Grief, a direct response to the loss of someone or something that we were deeply connected to, can be complex (and may be long-lasting). Waves of grief can show up anytime, and when they do, your aching heart may feel clenched. In the moment, stay with the feeling and put one or both hands in the center of the chest. Feel the warmth of your hands, and then try this practice.

- Slowly inhale up from the belly into the heart and exhale slowly, letting your chest ribs soften.

- To help the exhale sink deeper, soothe yourself by making a low *ooooo* tone (like the sound of the word *smooth*), letting it vibrate deep in the center of your body. Like humming, this sound helps to activate the vagus nerve, which soothes the heart.

- Stay with this as long as it feels nourishing, and allow yourself to feel whatever is present around what you're grieving.

- Now say to yourself, "May I give myself the compassion I need." Or try Heart-Centered Breath (page 151).

Fatigue or Exhaustion

You may feel depleted from unconsciously pushing yourself beyond your limits or having too many responsibilities. The restriction of the inhale (oxygen intake) and not fully exhaling (carbon dioxide buildup) can result in fatigue. Prolonged fatigue can eventually lead to burnout. Take time to restore your energy level with practices that recalibrate the in and out flow.

- Begin with an even-paced breathing of inhaling for 4 counts as you expand from your abdomen to your lower rib cage to your chest and exhaling for 4 counts. Gently move your body or spine as you breathe. Repeat 5 to 10 breath cycles throughout the day.

- To expand your breath and mental focus, try Box Breathing (page 205): Inhale for 4 counts, hold for 4, exhale for 4, hold for 4. Repeat 5 to 10 breath cycles twice a day.

- For a deeper refresher, stand for a minute and do Swinging Arms (page 170), then lie down on your back on a comfortable surface. Practice the Circle of Breath (page 126) to open the even flow of the in and out breaths and balance your energy level and your nervous system for 5 to 10 minutes.

Under Pressure

You have a deadline to meet for work, a school assignment, or an important event. You desperately need a break but don't have time to stop. Chances are, your nervous system is in the stress response, which means your breathing is tight and shallow and your body is starving for oxygen. Allow yourself 3 minutes (you can always take 3 minutes!) to calm, energize, and clear your mind with this rejuvenating exercise:

- Minute 1: Stand and shake out your body (this is a mini version of the Shaking practice on page 168). Make an *ah* sound as you exhale now and then to release the holding of tension.

- Minute 2: Now with your knees still soft and bouncing lightly, tap your body with relaxed hands—arms, chest, rib cage, lower back, hips, legs, head, or wherever it feels good to tap.

- Minute 3: Next, sit in a chair with your hands on your thighs. Breathe through your nose and flex your spine and rib cage forward on the inhale, slightly arching, and rounding back on the exhale, with your shoulders, jaw, and neck relaxed. Rock back and forth on your sit bones (see Rocking Spine, page 91).

- Stretch and move your body any way that feels good. Now breathe easy, slow, and steady and carry on!

Box Breathing

Also known as square breathing, this technique is used to deepen and slow the breath for better focus while staying calm and present. It is widely known to be the go-to practice of the Navy SEALs.

» Inhale for 4 counts, letting your breath start low in the abdomen and lower ribs, then filling up to the top of your lungs, just under your collarbone.

» Hold the air in for 4 counts, feeling your lungs filled with air.

» Exhale, emptying the air out of your lungs for 4 counts.

» Hold the air out for 4 counts. Repeat for 5 minutes or until you feel more focused and calm.

4-7-8 Breath

This yogic breath technique creates a deep level of relaxation, slowing the rate of breathing by holding the inhale and doubling the length of the exhale. It has been shown to be effective in relieving anxiety and also in helping people fall asleep.

» Lightly touch your tongue to the spot behind your front teeth.

» Exhale and let the air fall out of your mouth/throat, making an *ah* sound.

» Inhale gently through your nose for 4 counts.

» Hold for 7 counts.

» Exhale and let the air flow all the way out through rounded lips, making a *whoosh* sound, for 8 counts.

» If any of the counts are difficult to reach, start the whole practice with one less count and work up to it. Repeat 4 times, twice a day.

COPING WITH EXTERNAL FORCES

Driven by our feelings and mental states, our inner world of emotions and beliefs is part of what affects our breath. There's also the physical world we live in, with its environmental forces and circumstances beyond our bodies that can affect our respiratory function and patterns of breathing. Your body automatically goes into a holding or shallow breathing pattern, for example, when it encounters anything toxic in the air, whether that's exhaust from motor vehicles or chemical or gas smells from industrial sites. These external elements can block our breath and disrupt physiological and nervous system balance. To safeguard us from toxins, our breathing restricts to prevent us from inhaling them in, another example of the wisdom of the breath.

The Cleansing Breath

Kapalabhati is the Sanskrit word for a yoga practice often called the Skull Shining breath (*kapala* means "skull," and *bhati* means "to shine"). The quick action of this breath is known to cleanse and detoxify your lungs and body. It also tones your diaphragm, improves digestion, and increases oxygen to the blood. Once you get the hang of it, you can do a few of these breaths anytime you're hit with toxins in the air. I was introduced to this practice in a Kundalini yoga class more than thirty years ago. It will now come to me as an automatic response if I walk by a bus or car letting out a big puff of exhaust or find myself in an area with heavy air pollution. In those moments, I do a round of 10 or more of these breaths to make sure I am not taking in the toxins too deeply. Become familiar with this practice by following the instructions below. Kapalabhati is best practiced sitting in a chair or cross-legged on the floor with a straight and soft spine and on an empty stomach (the strong in-and-out movement of the abdomen can interfere with digestion. Wait a couple of hours if you have just eaten a full meal.)

Start at a slow pace and build up to about 1 exhale per second. Once it becomes easy and comfortable, you can double it to 2 breaths per second. If you get light-headed, agitated, or tense, try fewer breaths and gently work your way up to a few more. A note of caution: Do not breathe in this way if you are pregnant or menstruating, or if you have high blood pressure, heart disease, or gastrointestinal issues.

- Start by putting your hand on your abdomen and inhaling slowly and as fully as is comfortable without pushing.

- Let the exhale fall out of your mouth slowly, and let the inhale naturally fill your lungs about three-quarters full.

- Begin exhaling short and quick bursts through the nose, feeling your abdomen draw in toward your spine as a natural reaction with each one. It's important to focus mostly on the active exhales, letting your inhales happen naturally as your belly expands. As your breath goes out, your diaphragm goes up and you expel the air out of the lungs.

- Try 5 breath cycles now: Put your hand over your navel. With every out breath, feel how your abdomen goes inward and naturally bounces back out on the inhale. On your next exhale, breathe through your nose.

- Rest and let your inhale flow in. Continue to let your breath come and go freely. Try 5 more breath cycles. What do you notice? A sensation of warmth? Tingly or buzzy? Energized?

- Practice 10 breath cycles, then rest and breathe naturally and observe the sensations in your body. Repeat 10 breath cycles 3 or 4 times, resting in between each cycle.

- Start your day with this cleansing breath bath to help you wake up, or practice at midday or before dinner to clear your lungs of stale air. Use a round of 10 cycles whenever you encounter any kind of toxic air.

Breathing with a Face Mask On

In the spring of 2020, at the onset of the COVID-19 pandemic, I started teaching online breathwork classes at a yoga studio in Portland, Oregon. I wanted to include a practice on how to breathe comfortably while wearing a protective mask. A practice developed by Patrick McKeown, clinical director of the Buteyko Clinic International and author of *The Oxygen Advantage*, was helpful. He explains that for many people, wearing a mask causes a tendency to breathe fast and shallow through the mouth. This can create a breathing pattern that's too rapid and too hard to alleviate a feeling of suffocation. The key is to breathe more efficiently through the nose and to lower your respiratory rate and tidal volume, the amount of air that moves in and out of your lungs with each breath cycle, getting good ventilation through the alveoli (the little air sacs in the lungs that oxygenate the blood) and to feel calm. Basically, that means slower and deeper breathing, lower in the lungs. This coherent way of breathing is always beneficial but can be especially calming when you're wearing a mask.

Based on McKeown's work, here is a list of suggestions for breathing while wearing a mask. This is what I share with my own breathwork students and clients:

- Breathe in and out through your nose.

- Breathe low and deep into a soft belly and lower ribs.

- Take your time with light, slow, easy breaths at a steady pace—nothing big or forceful.

- Take in about 30 percent less breath than you normally would. It's okay to feel a little hungry for air. This is actually more efficient and improves the saturation of oxygen in your blood.

- It takes some getting used to because most of us are used to taking in too much air, too fast. If you start to feel anxious, relax and take in what feels comfortable at a slower pace.

BREATH FOR TRAUMA SUPPORT

Trauma takes many different forms and is experienced to varying degrees. I describe trauma with a simple definition used in a type of therapy called Somatic Experiencing, developed by Peter A. Levine, PhD: "Any experience that is too much, too fast, and too soon." There's no time for the nervous system to process what happened; trauma lies beyond the capacity to cope. When we get traumatized, our ability to notice what we are feeling in our body and emotions decreases because we are in the hyperarousal part of the brain, triggered by the sympathetic nervous system (SNS). Since the survival brain connects with the physical body whether we're fighting, fleeing, or freezing, we can't simply think our way out of trauma. We can, however, find release through connection with the body. Just the act of paying attention to yourself in a mindful way, including bringing awareness to the breath, can help. The awareness can take you out of the survival response in the brain stem, into the rational thinking part of the brain, the prefrontal cortex, where you can choose how you want to respond rather than giving in to a knee-jerk reaction. Participating in body-centered activities, such as yoga, qigong, dance, and walking, as well as doing deep-breathing exercises, has been shown to help regulate our internal states and reconnect the mind and body. When you feel present, centered, and clear in your mind, you know that the connection is restored. Even in the midst of trauma, conscious breathing, depending on the rate and depth, can bring us back to the present moment. (Note, however, that deep levels of trauma require specific treatment with a skilled trauma therapist.)

The counterbalance to "too much, too fast, and too soon" would be "less, slower, and more mindful." Hum and a Hug (page 64) is a practice I use to support those who need to gently open the flow of breathing and settle the nervous system. Feeling hand contact and the vibration of the hum sound, followed by sensing the movement of the inhale slowly entering the rib cage and arms, is an effective way to connect the body and mind while activating the vagus nerve and balancing the brain. Hum for at least 6 counts and rest at the bottom of the exhale, allowing the inhale to flow in easily and comfortably full when it's ready. Self-Compassion Breath (page 144) is also helpful when a trauma or intense stress is causing an inner struggle and a lack of self-support.

BREATHPLAY CORNER

Finding creative and fun ways to use conscious breathing are limitless and at the same time can relax and stimulate our brain as the nervous system calms and balances. A client of mine who was a musician and music producer helped me realize this a few years ago.

He would come in for a breath session for inspiration and would leave with one every time. Explore the following practices that combine breath with activities that help you to be present, while balancing your nervous system and giving your brain some playtime.

Doodling with the Breath

Just like regular doodling or coloring are relaxing, here, let your breath guide your doodle. Take a moment and notice how your breathing feels. Put your pen, pencil, paintbrush, color markers, etc., on a piece of paper. To get started, move your pen in one direction with your inhale and move it another with your exhale without trying to change your breath and see how long each line is. This is a breathing exploration, just to be curious and play. It can become a relaxing breath practice and spark creativity. As you continue breathing, let your pen move in different shapes and lengths, waves, spirals, angles, circles, squiggles, etc., one way on the inhale and another way on the exhale. Don't think; just see what happens.

Some ideas to help balance: If you would like to calm down, draw a longer line with a longer exhale. If you find yourself inhaling into your upper chest, draw a line downward or sideways as you inhale to illustrate bringing your breath lower to move the belly or rib cage. Or forget all that and surprise yourself as you draw a line on the in-breath and one on the out-breath. A slow and steady rhythm is nice for relaxation or you can play with different rhythms.

Ball Toss Breath

As Bessel van der Kolk encourages the use of rhythmic activities to regulate the nervous system and brain function with clients (tossing a ball back and forth, bouncing on a Pilates ball, drumming or dancing to music), besides bouncing on the big ball, I have been playing with tossing a ball from one hand to the other with a breathing rhythm and have also found it to support present moment focus.

Here are two exercises to try. Practice each for 3 to 10 minutes.

- **To calm and focus:** Tossing a ball from one hand to the other (easy rhythm)—right, left, right, left = one, two, three, four (4 counts on inhale through nose)—then repeat back and forth 4 times for the exhale through the mouth (more space to learn to let the air out at first). However, breathing out through the nose works well, too.

- **For more energy:** At a faster pace, toss two counts (right, left) and inhale, and two counts (right, left) and exhale. You could also lob the ball from one hand up in the air and catch it with the other. Inhale when you lob it up and exhale when it lands in the other hand. The higher you lob, the longer it expands the inhale. The exhale is just letting go—*ha*—when you catch it.

Laugh to Breathe, Live to Laugh

If you could put one breath-related practice at the top of your coping kit, make it laughter! As a way of breathing, laughter is one of the most powerful and natural forces we have within us. It is a gift of our shared humanity—we all feel the same when we do it. Laughter is contagious, in health-giving ways, helping us bond with others by making us feel unguarded and relaxed with each other in the moment. As a natural pain reliever, laughter releases endorphins, the brain's feel-good chemicals, while also decreasing the production of stress hormones. It also enhances your intake of oxygen and improves your cardiovascular system by stimulating the heart and lungs, clearing your lungs of stale air by exercising your breathing muscles. Specifically, when you laugh, you're loosening your diaphragm and dropping your breath lower to the abdominal area. Together, the benefits of laughter enhance your immune response. Reflect on how you can bring more laughter into your life, at least once a day, in any of the following ways:

- You know the type of humor you like. Find movies or videos that make you laugh. Collect them in a digital file that you can access easily.

- Call a friend you love to laugh with and take a break with them each day. I have my siblings and a couple of friends I will call if I need some of that feel-good relief.

- Join a Laughter Yoga class. (That's right—it's a thing.)

FOCUSING BREATH PRACTICES FOR CHILDREN

Children have had less time to form habitual patterns of tension and survival responses that create restricted breathing and are generally more open to learning breathing skills for support in a challenging situation.

Your first instinct in wanting to utilize the breath might be to say, "Take a deep breath," but when they are agitated, it could end up being a quick sharp inhale, feeding the stress response. A better message is to acknowledge that everyone—yourself included—should try to exhale to calm down, then take a breath. Demonstrating with a sigh or blowing the air out with pursed lips is a great place to start.

PRACTICE
Bedtime Breathing

This practice is one I've suggested to clients whose children have trouble settling down at bedtime. Honestly, it can also help anytime you want to turn on the relaxation response, instill calm, and impart a sense of safety.

» Start by focusing on letting the air out. Bring attention to the next exhale (children will inhale however much they need to) with a long *ah* sound through the mouth. The sound and volume on the *ah* can be however feels good or comfortable. Allow the child to have fun with the sound, which can be very freeing. Then inhale slowly and easily through the nose. Repeat 5 to 10 times or until there's an easy balance of the inhale and the exhale.

» Rest and feel easy breathing. Ask the child to put one hand on their belly and the other hand on their caregiver's belly. The adult will inhale and let their belly gently expand and soften back in with the exhale, so that the child's hand can feel the out-and-in movement and then follow the movement in their own body with the hand on their belly.

» Once they catch on to the coordination, place a stuffed animal (one with a little weight, or use a bean bag) on the child's belly and have them imagine giving it a little ride up with the inhale and down with the exhale. This turns into rocking the animal to sleep with the rise-and-fall movement. The pacing should be slow and easy, until the child is calm and ready to go to sleep.

» You can also add counting breaths to this, for example, inhaling for 2 or 3 counts and exhaling for 2 or 3 counts. Or count animal names instead of seconds, such as breathe in—*one turtle* (rabbit, froggy, doggy, etc.), *two turtles, three turtles*—breathe out: *one turtle, two turtles,* etc. The pacing can vary, as a child's breathing rate is generally faster than an adult's. The main point is to take it slow and steady.

Bumblebee Breath

This breath practice originates from a yoga technique called Bhramari breathing (*bhramari* is the Sanskrit term for "bee") and involves humming with the mouth closed on the exhale, mimicking the sound of a bumblebee. This works well when transitioning from a high level of energy to a more focused activity. This is a good practice for anyone, not just children.

» If the children are comfortable, ask them to close their eyes, which can add another level of focus. Otherwise, you can suggest that they look at the floor.

» When they're sitting comfortably, have them gently place the tips of their index fingers in their ears.

» Breathing through the nose, ask them to inhale easily and hum quietly as the exhale flows out. The whole face will feel as if it's buzzing, moving, vibrating; some kids say that the noise inside sounds much louder than the noises of the other kids doing the same thing.

» Try playing with the sound, imagining the bee flying around and making the sound louder and softer as it gets closer and farther away. Practicing for 2 to 5 minutes is usually all you need. Then rest and breathe easy and naturally. Ask the child to notice how they feel after the exercise and tell you what feels different.

Smell the Rose,
Blow Out the Candle

This is basically rounded or pursed-lip breathing with an image to play with.

» Have the child hold their index finger up to their nose, visualizing that it's a rose and taking in its fragrance with a long, slow inhale through the nose (putting an essential oil, like lavender, on the finger can help).

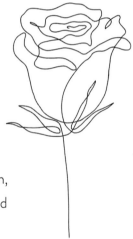

» Next, they can imagine their finger as a candle and pretend to blow it out with a controlled, steady stream of air, so they feel the breath on their fingertip. They will repeat this for 2 to 5 minutes. This teaches them to inhale slow and deep and exhale steady and completely. (Some teachers use this as a way to calm down an out-of-control classroom, practicing it until all the children have settled and slowed down, which can take 5 to 20 breath cycles or more.)

We are part of a universe that expands and
contracts in a dancing, pulsing movement
of life energy, a breathing relationship.

—MARGARET TOWNSEND

7

Breathing in Partnership

The Shared Experience of Breath

Opening up with breathwork allows you to become acquainted with yourself in a more conscious way. But did you know you can also broaden the experience of breathwork to enrich your relationships with others? Breathing together—whether with another person or in a group, as in a breathwork class—is powerful. The feeling of connection, of breathing in harmony, can also strengthen your commitment to the practice. In teaching breathwork classes, I often witness a greater sense of commonality and trust between students at the end of a group session as the breath frees up deeply held tensions in the body and mind. Sharing with each other after breathing together often awakens the component of compassion, our common humanity, by allowing us to appreciate the honesty and vulnerability in one another.

DEEPENING OUR RELATIONSHIPS BY WAY OF THE BREATH

Breathwork can enhance your relationship with a romantic partner, family member, friend, or colleague. In a romantic partnership, breathing together can strengthen your bond as a couple, offering a level of connection and intimacy that can't always be achieved with words. How? When we are relaxed and calm, we feel safe, connected, and engaged with each other thanks to the vagus nerve. As breathwork releases the "feel-good" chemicals, it makes connecting on a physical level more satisfying and heightens physical sensations.

Breathing in communion is a chance for transparency, allowing you to see through thoughts you may have about each other in order to share honestly with kindness with your partner in the practice. It allows you to recognize your commonality. We sometimes forget, or maybe aren't even aware, that the people we are in relationships with tighten their breath and body when they are feeling fear and anxiety just as we do. Bringing awareness to this truth fosters understanding and compassion, when we may be focusing only on behavior or defenses during or after an argument, for example.

When you experience the power of conscious breathing, you can connect intimately to what is meaningful to you and to the essence of who you truly are. Intimacy with another then becomes a welcome adventure of openness and bonding. The following practices support you in being with another person in an integrated way—body, heart, and mind. Each of these practices can be done as a couple or with anyone you want to explore having a better relationship with. Can you stay open to another person beyond what you think or know about them? Let the breath take you there.

To begin, both of you will set an intention for each practice, whether it's to feel closer, alleviate tension between you, or be open to more conscious and effective communication. As you listen to the other person's intention, let yourself stay present to what they want rather than think about or analyze their intention. If you lose focus or your mind wanders, keep coming back to your initial intention of being and breathing with this person so you can share the benefits.

Breathing with a Partner

Awareness in these practices will first help connect you to yourselves so you can both stay present with each other. Start with the following steps before moving on to any of the other practices.

» Sit together and close your eyes.

» Start by finding your own breath moving in your body.

» Get in touch with what you would like to receive from partnered breathing. Speak that out loud to each other.

» Notice how you feel when hearing your partner's words. Any tension in your body? In your breath? If yes, soften your belly to receive the breath and help you be more receptive to them.

» Now listen as you keep coming back to your gentle flow of breath.

» Take turns sharing what you feel.

PRACTICE
Back-to-Back Breathing

The purpose of this partner practice is to experience a wordless way to pay attention, listen, and respond.

» Find a comfortable way to sit—on the floor with cushions or stools, or on two chairs side by side with your backs touching in the natural places they do without leaning into each other. Feel the closeness and warmth of your backs touching.

» Notice your breath moving inside your body and the quality of it: tight, easy, deep, shallow, fast, slow?

» Now become aware of your partner's breath. What can you feel about their breathing pattern? Try to be aware of your breathing together without changing anything, creating a dialogue with your breathing backs. Let your breath be yours and theirs be theirs. What is that like? Stay with that for a few minutes.

» Now bring your breath rhythms together. Notice what it takes for you both to allow this to happen nonverbally: agreement, understanding, and accommodation. Stay with that for a few minutes.

» To finish, come back and find your own rhythm and way of breathing as you keep contact with your backs and notice the connection with yourself and each other.

» When you're ready, turn and face each other in silence and notice if you feel a difference in your energy or breath. When you're ready, share your experience with each other.

Full-Circuit Breath

This practice creates a circuit (like one that carries an electrical current) of breath that flows between two people. It can be done with anyone you want to create a stronger connection with.

The intention for this practice is to appreciate your partner and focus on what you love about them. There's always a mix of good and difficult feelings in every relationship. Allow any other feelings that are present to be here as well and keep coming back to your intention.

» Sit comfortably facing each other without touching. Close your eyes and acknowledge to yourself that there are times you may have struggled with love and acceptance for yourselves and each other.

» Become aware of all the love that's right below the surface. It's there, like the sun behind the clouds. Stay there for 2 to 3 minutes, or however long you need.

» Open your eyes and make eye contact. If it feels too intense, focus on just one of your partner's eyes.

» Breathe through your nose, and synchronize your breath so that you both breathe in at the same time and breathe out at the same time at a slow, easy pace. Try a count of 4 in and 4 out for 3 to 5 breaths or however long it takes to feel in sync.

» Next, keeping the same rhythm, take turns so that one person inhales as the other exhales. Find a gentle breathing rhythm together with that pattern, like riding a seesaw. The person exhaling will send the feeling of love to the other partner in whatever aspect feels sincere, whether it's compassion, gratitude, or kindness. The other will inhale and receive this loving breath from their partner and for themselves. As you exhale, send what you're feeling out from your chest, from your eyes to your partner. You don't have to say it, just feel it and send it. You may get out of sync with the breathing, emotions arising, your mind wandering, or a break in eye contact (it's okay to take a break, but do come back to it). Keep returning to the breath and eye contact with each other as much as you can.

» Stay with this for 5 to 10 minutes, or longer. Then close your eyes. Breathe now at an easy, natural rhythm and feel what you feel.

» When you're ready, open your eyes and talk with each other about your experience.

PRACTICE
Side-by-Side Breathing

For this practice, you're experiencing the power of gentle conscious connected breathing together (see Circle of Breath, page 126) to open and deepen on your own but with each other. Your intention may be to calm down together to gain more understanding for each other, to listen better by responding to the other's needs, or just to take time to connect with your breath rather than words. Just breathe together freely and see where it takes you.

» Lie down side by side on a comfortable surface, either on a mat on the floor or on a bed or outside on the grass—wherever feels best. Breathe in a gentle connected flow (see Circle of Breath, page 126) through an open throat and mouth, with a relaxed jaw, allowing the inhale and exhale to flow into each other like water in a waterwheel, flowing in and falling out. If it feels uncomfortable to breathe through the mouth, continue through the nose (keep your throat open and jaw soft). Start slowly with a count of 3 or 4 for the inhale and let the exhale fall freely until it lands.

» Once you get the rhythm, let go of the counting and just feel the breath flowing in and falling out in an easy comfortable rhythm. Breathe, without touching each other, for 5 minutes, then hold hands (if it's comfortable to do so) and continue breathing for 5 minutes.

» As this gets more comfortable and familiar, play with extending the time to 10 minutes without touching and 10 minutes holding hands. Stay open and respectful of yourself and each other if either of you needs to shift positions. It's okay if you pause or drift; keep coming back to your gently flowing breath.

» Let go of your hands. Rest and let your breath flow through your nose. Let the ground hold you for a few minutes or until you're ready to move.

» Stretch your body any way that feels good—arms up over your head, through your legs, or bringing your knees in to your chest to stretch your lower back—before sitting up. Take turns sharing your experience with each other, speaking and listening openly.

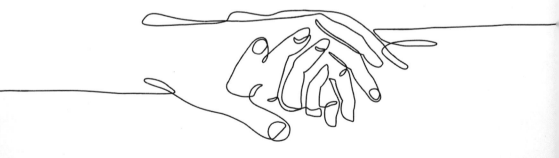

Howie and Jana had been married for several years; they had a strong relationship. In recent years, however, as their lives had become busier and more stressful, tension had built up between them. On top of their separate jobs, they owned a company together. They came to me hoping to find a way back to an easy and relaxed connection. They started with the Back-to-Back Breathing (page 224), and acknowledged how sweet it was to sit and feel their backs touching and each other's breath moving. Both shared that at first their breath was smaller; Jana noticed that she held her breath to feel Howie's breath. They were amazed when their breath started naturally moving in sync, just happening together. At the end, when they came back to their own breath, Howie observed that his breath was slower and easier. Jana said she could feel her inhale starting lower and more in her side rib cage area. Next, they went into the Full-Circuit Breath practice (page 226). They began playing on their own, holding hands, palm to palm, eventually moving their hands in a circle as they breathed. They said it was like passing a ball of love back and forth with their breath and admitted that it had been a long time since they focused on each other. They both felt closer from the experience. Howie and Jana later reported that throughout the busy days that followed, they felt extra close and connected, with an intuitive sense between them that fostered easier communication.

BREATHING TOGETHER IN
THE WORK ENVIRONMENT

Beyond teaching breathwork to individuals and small groups, I have worked with companies at annual retreats and team-building meetings. Even though this idea is outside the traditional workplace culture, it can be a benefit for any team of colleagues. At the end of our sessions, I suggest coworkers continue with this simple practice at regular meetings throughout the year:

- Sit together for a moment at the beginning of the meeting so that each person can find and feel the breath moving somewhere in their body.

- "Take 5" together (quietly inside): 5 breaths for 5 counts on the inhale and 5 counts on the exhale (4 counts is okay, too). This gives everyone time to:

  - Settle as a group.

  - Get clear of the intention, goal, and ideas for the meeting.

  - Find the willingness to listen to each other.

  - During the meeting, keep coming back to your breathing to accomplish the intention!

BREATHING INTO OUR
RELATIONSHIP WITH NATURE

In many ways, the greatest partnership we can cultivate through the breath is our relationship with nature. Being out in nature with plants, trees, flowers, air, water, and animals can bring us into a more quiet mind, calm our nervous system, and slow our breathing. There's only the simple being with our senses. Using conscious breathing can enhance this experience.

In his book *Stillness Speaks*, spiritual teacher and author Eckhart Tolle writes, "You can reconnect with nature in the most intimate and powerful way by becoming aware of your breathing and learning to hold your attention there."

The plant world participates with us in the process of respiration. Just as we inhale oxygen and exhale carbon dioxide, plants take in carbon dioxide (and carbon emissions) and release oxygen through the process of photosynthesis, which is essential for all life. It's no wonder that our trees and forests are called the lungs of the earth! When we consciously engage our breath with the plant kingdom's breath, we can experience how we give to and receive from each other. Become aware of this intimate and powerful cycle of life, the relationship you share as you exchange the flow of life-force energy with nature in this way. As you consciously breathe with the following practice, know that you are not separate from all of nature. Rather, you are contributing to your own well-being and every living being on the planet.

Nature Breathing

This practice is rooted in the same Full-Circuit Breath (page 226) you would do with a partner—giving and receiving. It can be a calming sitting or walking mindful meditation as well as an expanded experience of consciousness anytime you're in nature, and want to slow down and relax your thinking mind and come back to the nature of yourself. If you're indoors, breathe with an indoor plant or when looking at trees or other plant life outside your window.

» Inhale and take in the life-sustaining oxygen the plant world is giving you. Exhale and give nature back the carbon dioxide it needs to live. Breathe in a circular way, receiving, giving, receiving, giving back.

» Stay with this steady flow of breathing for at least 10 minutes, or however long you want to. The longer you practice, the deeper you go. As you breathe, look, feel, and listen to the sacred natural world around you with which you're now connecting.

VARIATION

» To express your gratitude, inhale the words *thank you* as you take in what nature is giving you. Exhale the words *for you* and give back as an act of compassion. Research shows that when we experience gratitude and compassion, our brain releases dopamine, serotonin, and oxytocin, chemicals that enhance pleasure and make us happy.

Expanding the Circle of Love

Breathing with this focus is a way to cultivate loving-kindness and to create a heartfelt, compassionate connection with others while having it for yourself as well. This practice was created as a way to expand your circle of caring and love.

» Sit comfortably and let your eyes close. Bring a hand to your chest as a reminder that you are bringing loving awareness to your experience.

» As you breathe in, become aware that your body is being nourished. When you breathe out, notice how your body can settle and be calmed. Then find the natural rhythm of the breath, nourishing and soothing. Stay with this for a few moments.

» You can let your hands relax in your lap with your palms facing up. Now think of someone you love. On your next exhale, send love and good wishes to that person from the center of your heart out through every cell of your body. Then inhale through every cell into your heart and receive love and good wishes.

» Continue for a few breaths, with love and warm wishes flowing out and back to you in a gentle, easy rhythm. Give, receive. Inhale, exhale.

» Now think of your friends and family. Exhale and send them love and good wishes out from your heart through your cells. Inhale and receive it through every cell to your heart. Stay here for a few breaths.

» Now bring to mind people you struggle with or have a difficult relationship with. Exhale and send them love and good wishes from your heart through every cell of your body. Inhale and receive love and warmth through every cell to your heart. Stay here for a few breaths. Breathing out love, breathing in love. Your heart knows that we all need and want love. Inhale, exhale.

» Extend your circle of connection to all people suffering on the planet. Exhale and send them love and good wishes from your heart out through every cell of your body. Inhale and receive love and good wishes in through every cell to your heart. Love and warmth flowing from your heart to others, returning back to you. Taking in, giving back. Inhale, exhale. Stay here for a few breaths.

» Now expand your awareness to all living beings on the planet. Exhale and send all beings love and good wishes from your heart out through every cell of your body. Inhale and receive love and good wishes in through every cell to your heart.

» Your wisdom of your heart knows that we all share the breath, that we are all connected. All breathing bodies, all breathing cells. Cells and bodies breathing love. Stay with this as long as you want to. Inhale love. Exhale love.

Breathing unites mind and body, gives access to the master controls of the involuntary nervous system. It's a practice. It's the constancy that produces dramatic changes.

—DR. ANDREW WEIL

8

Building Your Breathwork Routine

Maintaining Your New Normal

I remember the moment when I realized that the perception of practice can evolve from something you "have to do" into something you "get to do." I was in the middle of sitting in silence, bringing awareness to my breath during my morning practice. As my breath flowed effortlessly, it spontaneously became an experience of deep calm and peace that filled my body and mind. I couldn't wait to feel that deep sense of well-being again and again! What I love about working with the breath is that it can support you in any moment and carry you throughout the day. There is a sense of empowerment when we know we have a practice to support and nourish ourselves with for the rest of our lives. It is my wish for you to know that your breath can give you this experience.

Think of a daily activity that's good for your well-being, a healthy habit that you miss when you aren't able to get to it. That's what the intention could be for making breathwork practice an essential part of your life. Your own breathwork journey is likely to evolve over time, adapting to natural changes and needs in your life. As you give yourself time to practice on a regular basis, your awareness of the breath will continue to develop.

Dr. Andrew Weil, founder and director of the Center for Integrative Medicine at the University of Arizona, emphasizes the importance of adhering to a regular breathwork routine. He suggests that repetitively using conscious breathing rhythms will gradually create change in the autonomic nervous system (ANS). According to Dr. Weil, "it is the regularity that produces changes, not intensity or how much in one day." Stay open. Find your willingness. Experiment with a variety of practices, letting your intuition guide you to a routine that works for you.

It can be challenging to find the discipline to begin and maintain a new practice. Maybe it seems like you don't have enough energy, or it's hard to slow down enough to follow through, or your mind is just too busy to make space for it.

ROUTINE ESSENTIALS

Putting together a breathwork routine—and committing to it—doesn't have to be complicated. When clients ask for advice, I usually encourage them to think in terms of three elemental parts, which I call the three Ps: presence, participation, and practice. It's an easy way to stay focused.

PRESENCE: Being present, or mindful in the moment, makes it possible to use the breath as a portal for transformation, meaning inner change. Think of it this way: You may get an invitation to an event that says "Your presence is requested." That language does not mean just your body. It speaks to every part of you. To receive the benefits of conscious breathing, your presence is not only *requested* but *required*. Breathwork connects you to and infuses the four levels of your self as a human being—the physical, emotional, mental, and spiritual—into an experience of feeling whole.

PARTICIPATION: Being actively committed to a breathwork practice expresses your willingness to build a relationship with the breath and a healthier life. This engagement with the process accesses the wisdom of your breath and energy to go where it's needed, to balance, heal, and rejuvenate on all levels. As you participate with it, welcome it.

PRACTICE: Because repatterning happens with repetition, a dedicated practice allows for a transformational experience that creates nourishing change. This is the way to gradually regulate your nervous system, so as you breathe freer, you feel freer inside your own body and mind. Choose practices that are enjoyable and meaningful to you and create a new normal for a life worth breathing.

CREATING YOUR PERSONAL PRACTICE

Having a breathwork practice is a gift to yourself—not only the gift of better health, but that of a physical feeling of spaciousness inside. Design your routine so that you look forward to receiving these gifts, like a mini vacation or inner spa time that you can work into your daily schedule. Give yourself this time to settle into your body, into your heart. Practice receiving and allowing with every inhale and exhale, taking in the good and softening into that. You are expanding your capacity to better tolerate stress and accept more life energy, more joy (from your endorphins), more presence, and, ultimately, more love.

To develop a schedule, set aside 10 to 60 minutes a day to practice, if you can; experiment to find the timing that works best for you, even if it's just 5 minutes to start. Some people practice at the same time every day, morning or evening. If your life is chaotic or you tend to feel scattered, it may make sense to choose a regular time. Starting your day with breathwork helps keep you more conscious of it all day. When you greet each morning with calming practices, you're better able to switch on and activate the relaxation response, which can help set the tone for the day and can help you bounce back more easily when stressful moments arise. Energetic practices can give you the boost you need to get going in the morning and to carry you through the day.

For others, being flexible about practice time allows them the freedom to work around their own schedules, including family and work. In those cases, dispersing individual practices throughout the day and evening is a better option.

If you plan to practice primarily at home, consider designating a special or sacred space for breathwork, a place where you can settle down and settle in. Your sacred space could be as simple as a chair and a side table with a candle or an object that's meaningful to you. Ideally, the spot will reflect the feeling that you want to have on the inside: calm, quiet, spacious (even if it's a small room), something that makes you exhale when you're there.

Find a spot with a comfortable temperature, a place to sit, room to stand and move, and a soft surface to lie down on. Keep a blanket and pillow(s) handy in case you need them. Add a few things that appeal to your senses, such as objects whose colors you like or fresh flowers; I often use a diffuser with essential oils. Think about whether you want ambient noise or music or complete quiet. Finally, make it a device-free zone. Give yourself the luxury of tech-free time, even if it's brief.

STRUCTURING YOUR PRACTICE: PUTTING IT ALL TOGETHER

Here is a list of the practices and suggestions for how you can use them. Not all practices work in the same way for everyone. Consider your preferences and choose accordingly. You may prefer counting, or paced, breathing exercises, for example, to give the mind something to focus on. Or you may be drawn to the chance to simply feel the free flow of breath in the body and keep your attention on the experience.

As you read through the combinations of exercises, know that there is overlap with the benefits that may seem contradictory. A relaxation practice and a movement or energizing practice can both give you more mental clarity, for example, because of the way breathwork balances your brain and nervous system, depending on your needs. I have watched students in class do the exact same exercise and feel completely different—one more relaxed because they started in stress mode and another who came in with fatigue becoming more alert and energetic. Each responded in the way their body needed for balance.

The following concepts are the three parts of a well-rounded practice: befriending the breath by coming into conscious relationship with it, then taking action to open up your breathing muscles and body to welcome a healthy breath, and finally using specific ways of breathing to regulate your system and deepen conscious awareness in response to your needs and inclination. Whether it's to start your morning or simply to meet your ever-changing needs, anytime is a good time to be aware and open your breath.

AWARENESS: Start with a practice that directs your attention to the breath.

OPENING UP: Choose one or more of the Breath and Body Openers on the following page.

BRINGING THE BREATH TO LIFE: Respond with any of the need-based practices, depending on where you feel an inner call for balance. Are you looking for relaxation, energy, clarity, openness, or self-compassion? Be creative and find what works.

TIP: With any practice, ease up on any forced or strained effort to pull the inhale in or push the exhale out. Remember, less can be better when you're breathing with tense muscles and a nervous system in stress mode.

PRACTICE GUIDELINES

PURPOSE	PRACTICES	HOW IT WORKS
AWARENESS	Take Your Seat (page 28); Discovering Your Breathing Spaces (page 30); Wake Awareness with a Rub (page 40)	Noticing breath, without changing it, begins to bring you into relationship with your breath, body, and mind.
BODY AND BREATH OPENERS	Wake Up the Respiratory Diaphragm (page 86); Wake Up the Belly (page 88); Wake Up the Pelvic Diaphragm (page 89); Rocking the Spine (page 91), sitting; Stretching to Make Space (page 92); Sitting Body Circles (page 95); Tuck and Rock (page 117), lying down; Twist and Roll (page 118), lying down	By opening up breath flow and the breathing spaces to help you feel and wake up your diaphragm and other breathing muscles in the neck, abdomen, spine, intercostals, and pelvis, allowing space for optimal breathing.
RELAXATION	Hum and a Hug (page 64); Freeing the Exhale (page 72); Coherent Breathing (page 122); Box Breathing (page 205); 4-7-8 Breath (page 206)	By stimulating the parasympathetic response through lengthening the exhale, inhaling lower, and slowing the pace of breathing to create an easy flow.
ENERGY	"Ha" Breath (page 164); Breath Ball (page 165); Shaking (page 168); Swinging Arms (page 170); Swinging Twists (page 172); Rhythmic Walking and Breathing (page 175); Breath Dance (page 176); Tap and Pat (page 179); Heart Wings (page 184)	By deepening and lengthening the inhale and increasing the breath pace. These practices combine synchronized movement and breath and help with circulation and connection with your body.

Every day. Tune in and wake up to your breath with these practices to create a habit of connecting with it throughout the day. When you're short on time, take a couple of minutes for each.

Every day. After breath awareness, notice any area of your breathing space that's not open or that feels tight, and do one or more of these first three opening practices that are related to the tight area. If your breath feels shallow overall, do the first three Wake Up practices together each time as a sequence, then lie down and explore diaphragmatic breathing for 3 more minutes. Explore any of the other ones that your body and breath needs or are drawn to, to enhance opening.

When your breath is shallow and tight, and you're looking to calm down, feel soothed, or gain mental clarity.

If you want more energy and to release tension in the body. Choose at least one each day or anytime you need it. Try them in the morning to wake up, midday to energize, or before dinner to rejuvenate, and revitalize.

PURPOSE	PRACTICES	HOW IT WORKS
SELF-COMPASSION	Self-Compassion Breath (page 144); Heart-Centered Breath (page 151)	By stimulating the PNS and vagus nerve through gentle compassionate words, voice, breath, touch—opening your heart and giving yourself the kindness and comfort you need.
DEEPER BREATH PROCESS	Circle of Breath (page 126)	By breathing at a gentle, connected pace to stimulate a balance between the parasympathetic system and the sympathetic nervous system for relaxed energy and deeper conscious awareness. This practice unwinds and softens holding patterns of contraction and helps to integrate the benefits of all other practices.
BREATHING IN RELATIONSHIP	Breathing with a Partner (page 224); Back-to-Back Breathing (page 224); Full-Circuit Breath (page 226); Side-by-Side Breathing (page 227)	By allowing you to connect with another person through the breath on another level, often beyond words.
GUIDED MEDITATIONS	Easing into Your Breath (page 34); Heart-Centered Breath (page 151); Nature Breathing (page 233); Expanding the Circle of Love (page 234)	By providing guided quiet time for letting the breath lead you to a deeper inner connection with yourself and the intention of each practice.

Anytime you're struggling emotionally or mentally, either with your inner critic or anything else, and you want to be more kind to yourself.

If you want to use your breathing to go deeper inside to connect with a stronger flow of breath and expand conscious awareness. Practice 2 times a week or up to every day, for 5 to 10 minutes (or a count of 50 to 100 breaths) at a time. You can also end your daily practice with 20 to 50 gentle connected breaths.

If there is a mutual desire to explore this level of breath together.

If you want to be enriched by one of the following practices. The longer you stay with these practices, the deeper they will take you into the experience and intention. Sitting or lying down, practice for 10 to 20 minutes, or longer if you want. (Sitting can keep you more alert.)

MORNING AND EVENING BREATH PRACTICES

As part of your breathwork practice, consider a routine that bookends each day, getting up from or settling into bed with a focus on the breath. The Morning Practice is what I do just after waking up, when I am still in bed. If you prefer getting out of bed to practice, you can lie on a mat on the floor.

PRACTICE
Morning Practice

While you're still in bed, tap into the flow of energy in your body by gently opening your breath and letting yourself become aware of your breath. The goal is to help awaken the body, clear any grogginess, and give you energy to face the day. This can take as few as 5 minutes or as many as 20 minutes, depending on how long you do the Heart-Centered Breath meditation (page 151).

» Notice any thoughts that start rushing in. Maybe you're planning the day ahead or mentally writing your to-do list for work. Whatever it is, instead of following the thoughts, choose yourself first and bring attention to your body. Stay with yourself in a mindful moment of just noticing what's here.

» Now find your breath. Shift from whatever position you woke up in to lie on your back. Rub your belly in a circle a few times, up the right side, then down the left. Rest your hands on your belly, allowing it to gently expand into your hands as you inhale for 5 to 10 breaths. Repeat by rubbing your upper abdomen (solar plexus) and then lightly pat your chest and ribs.

» Become aware of what you want to be open to today. Put your hands on your chest and do the Heart-Centered Breath meditation (page 151). Let intentional or kind words come, or just feel the energy of your breath grounding you in your heart. Repeat for about 5 minutes or until you feel good and present with the intention.

» Now just stretch in any way that feels good to you. Imagine how a cat stretches and allow yourself to luxuriate in that slow and long movement. Notice how that opened your breathing.

» Finally, wake up the breath and spine with Tuck and Rock (page 117) and/or Twist and Roll (page 118), which I practice regularly. (You can also do this lying on the floor, if getting out of bed helps you stretch more fully.)

If you have time, consider the categories beginning on page 244, and try an awareness practice (sitting quietly); a body and breath opener; standing and moving with breath; or a calming and centering practice like Coherent Breathing (page 122) or Circle of Breath (page 126) for 20 or more cycles. Give yourself a word of kindness. Enjoy your day!

Evening Practice

Before you turn in for the night, it's important to calm the body, unwind, and breathe for better sleep. To transition from a fast-paced movement throughout the day to a more mellow rhythm, try a slow breathing and movement practice like Breath Ball (page 165). The calming, soothing breath encourages relaxation and rest.

» Begin with a gentle Circle of Breath practice (page 126) for 5 to 10 minutes, as a mini breath bath. You can do this in the bathtub or lying down on the bed.

» Before you get under the covers, lie on your bed so that your ankles hang off, to enable full range of motion when you circle your ankles. Bring your arms over your head. (It might help to lie perpendicular to the headboard, so that your ankles can hang off one side and your upper arms easily hang above your head.) After a day of habitual ways of holding the body, it's good to stretch out and elongate the rib cage, the whole body, and the breath.

» Inhaling, slowly flex your toes up on both feet for a count of 4, then exhale as you slowly point your toes for a count of 4. Continue slowly flexing for 4 and pointing for 4, repeating the full cycle 10 times. (Breathe to 5 counts if that feels better; find the count rhythm that feels slow and easy for you.) This will activate the pressure points around your ankles and feet and help with relaxation and sleep.

» Next, circle your ankles 20 times in one direction and 20 times in the other direction. Let your breath flow into your soft belly.

» Stretch in any way that feels good to you. Try stretching your arms and legs open and out as long as you can; rounding your back and arching your back; and/or stretching the sides of your ribs by bringing your knees to one side and your arms and head to the other side.

» When you're ready, get under the covers and give your body to the bed and your head to the pillow. Let the bed hold you. Give each exhale to gravity, to the bed, and to the ground, and let your breath gently flow into and soften your neck, shoulders, spine, ribs, hips, and limbs. If you feel any point of tension, let your exhale carry it down, and lay it on the bed to rest and be held. Let your breath find your belly and settle there in a gentle movement for the night.

Note: If you have trouble falling asleep, try 4-7-8 Breath (page 206). Repeat 4 times. Or count each exhale (slow and gentle) like the old recommendation of counting sheep. Notice how soon you drift off.

The longer
you stay
with a
breath practice,
the deeper
the benefit.

BE YOUR OWN BREATHWORK GUIDE

It's possible to use any of the practices in this book to make your own audio breathwork practice guide in your own voice. Read the practices or guided meditations aloud and record yourself on your phone so you can follow along and have the practice with you anytime. It is very powerful to hear your own voice guiding you and giving you support. In particular, talking yourself through the Circle of Breath connected breathing practice (page 126) is potent, as the process can take you into deeper breathing with your own voice. As you record, speak in the way you like to be spoken to, paying attention to your tone and volume. Or imagine yourself speaking to someone you love and care about. Remember that a soft, gentle voice helps soothe the nervous system. Add any words that have meaning for you. Or consider reading a quote or poem from this book—or anything that inspires you.

SAMPLE DAILY ROUTINES

Generally, my daily routine includes the Morning and Evening practices (as described on pages 248–251) in bed every day. Once I'm out of bed, I sit for a few minutes (or longer, depending on my schedule) in breath awareness before moving into the connected Circle of Breath practice (page 126). Then I may do some breath-opening and movement practices, or disperse them throughout my day. For example, I regularly do the Shaking (page 168) and Tap and Pat (page 179) practices throughout the day. I also take a rhythmic walk outside every day.

SHORTER ROUTINES

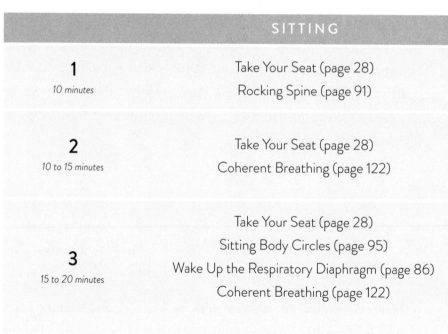

SITTING	
1 *10 minutes*	Take Your Seat (page 28) Rocking Spine (page 91)
2 *10 to 15 minutes*	Take Your Seat (page 28) Coherent Breathing (page 122)
3 *15 to 20 minutes*	Take Your Seat (page 28) Sitting Body Circles (page 95) Wake Up the Respiratory Diaphragm (page 86) Coherent Breathing (page 122)

Each of the following routines is a sample of how you can create your own routine using the Practice Guidelines chart on pages 244-247. Feel free to mix and match the practices in any way that feels good to you.

STANDING	LYING DOWN
Circle of Breath (page 126)	
Breath Ball (page 165)	
Shaking (page 168)	Tuck and Rock (page 117)
Tap and Pat (page 179)	Circle of Breath (page 126)
Swinging Arms (page 170)	

LONGER ROUTINES

	SITTING
1 *30 minutes*	Take Your Seat (page 28) Freeing the Exhale (page 72) Wake Up the Respiratory Diaphragm (page 86) Wake Up the Belly (page 88) Rocking Spine (page 91)
2 *40 to 60 minutes*	Take Your Seat (page 28) Hum and a Hug (page 64) Wake Up the Respiratory Diaphragm (page 86) Wake Up the Belly (page 88) Wake Up the Pelvic Diaphragm (page 89) Stretching to Make Space (page 92)

VARIED ROUTINE

	MORNING
Throughout the Day	Discovering Your Breathing Spaces (page 30) Rocking Spine (page 91) Swinging Twists (page 172)

STANDING	LYING DOWN
Shaking (page 168) Breath Ball (page 165)	Rub belly, ribs, chest Circle of Breath (page 126) Rest
Tap and Pat (page 179) Swinging Twists (page 172)	Twist and Roll (page 118) Circle of Breath (page 126) Rest

AFTERNOON	EVENING
Shaking (page 168), tapping chest with long *ahhhhh* sounds	Twist and Roll (page 118), lying on the floor Circle of Breath (page 126)

I encourage clients to create individualized routines depending on their needs, schedules, and lifestyles. Two of my clients integrated the following breathwork practice programs into their lives based on what they learned from our sessions.

Dana

Dana, a single mom of two preschoolers, wanted a practice to keep her grounded and centered. She created one that utilizes conscious breathing throughout the day.

» To open her body and spine, she starts with sitting spinal flexes and lying-down twisting.

» For energy and settling, she does shaking, swinging, and tapping practices. To calm herself, she uses her hands to rub and contact her breathing space and then extends her exhale longer than the inhale, sometimes with paced breathing and sometimes focusing on the exhale with the hum or zzzzz sounds and then lets the inhale come in when it does. She also combines rhythmic breathing while she rocks in a chair or swings in a hammock.

» At the end of her day, she will lie on her back with her legs up against the wall and do 20 ankle circles in both directions while breathing in an easy flow with her hands on her belly. She then does about 10 minutes of the Circle of Breath practice (page 126).

Leslie

During the earliest days of the COVID-19 pandemic, Leslie actually enjoyed the quieter and slower lifestyle. When the restrictions from the lockdown began to lift, she began having severe anxiety, to her surprise. Making decisions became difficult, and she worried about the future. She already practiced yoga, but she wanted to find ways to explore how to use the breath to help calm her and relieve her constant anxiety. After her first session, she reported feeling free from anxiety for the first time in months. Incorporating the following practices worked best for her in a regular morning practice.

» Hum and a Hug (page 64), patting the chest

» Wake Up the Respiratory Diaphragm (page 86) and Wake Up the Belly (page 88), using your hands to help feel the breath

» Rocking Spine (page 91)

» Twist and Roll (page 118)

» Soft pursed-lip breathing, wind tunnel breathing (like blowing out a candle)

» Gentle Circle of Breath (page 126), 5 minutes

Breath Is

Even when we hold against it because we are afraid of
*   where it will take us,*
to our feelings—
our deep discomfort,
our anxieties,
our fears,
how we have always known ourselves . . .
flawed, ugly, abnormal,
to our depth—
our out-of-the-boxness,
our freedom.
It waits,
this nourishing formless movement of life
this nothingness,
this everything
right here,
always,
for us to turn back to
so it can carry us to remembering
what we forgot—
the wisdom,
the truth
of what we can trust.

—MARGARET TOWNSEND

Coming Full Circle

Part III extends our own inner experience of breathing to bring it in communion with life around us. Wherever you go, it's right there with you. It's there to help you be with anything and everything. Consciously, you can use it as a resource, or unconsciously, it can get tangled with all those stressful emotions and thoughts, as you have noticed.

The diagram on the following page represents you inside your circle of your life—with your issues, circumstances, relationships, desires, and needs. This activity is intended to give you a moment to reflect on what you received from the book. For example, here are some things you might want to think about: Are there any ways it has helped create change in your breath or awareness of the breath? How? What do you feel you've learned from this book that you want to take with you and nurture to support you in your daily life?

1) Sit with your hands in your lap, palms open and facing up, breathing gently.

2) Reflect on and answer the following questions by drawing or writing on the diagram or another paper.

Draw or write within the body chart to show how any aspect of your breathing (awareness, pace, depth, space, location in your spaces, thoughts, feelings about them) is different now at the end of the book than it was before you picked it up. This is not about having completed all the practices by now; this is an evaluative awareness question. Change

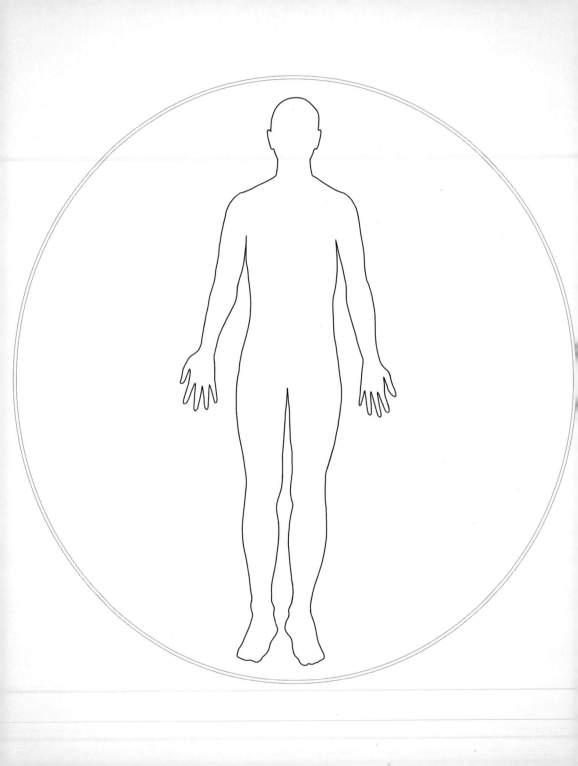

Change happens from simply noticing, from mindful awareness. This reflection is to invite you to check in and see if anything from this book—information, practices, new perspectives—created any change with your breath or in yourself. It may have, it may not have. Take your time and feel your breath and body now. Notice any way that you feel different or any change from noticing and consciously experiencing your breath. How is it different from the chart in the first chapter?

Draw and/or write answers to these questions around the body chart within the circle: What are you taking with you and bringing into your breathing circle of life? Any new thoughts, perceptions, or ideas, a new or surprising experience, a practice that turned out to be particularly impactful for you, a new question or curiosity about breath that you didn't have before?

What do you notice that happens all by itself inside when you hear that your breath is here for you, that life is here for you? There might be a "yeah, but . . ." thought, or it could create a reassuring feeling. Write or draw anything that occurs to you in your body or mind when you hear or read that. If there is a little argument, breathe with it! If it feels good, breathe with it! If it's neutral, yep, breathe with it! Stay curious and keep going: Stay with your practice because your breath is with you until your last exhale. Befriend it, give it space, and it will give you a rich life!

Afterword

Let's end the book with three breaths together to begin our next chapter:

Put one or both hands on your chest.

Inhale and hold it and say a wish or prayer of peace from yourself to yourself. Exhale and let it sink deeper into your heart.

Inhale and hold it and let a person or people come to mind and say a wish or prayer of peace for them.

Exhale and send that out to them.

Inhale and hold it and say a wish or prayer of peace to the planet and all beings. Exhale and send it out.

May we remember that we are all connected together in breath.

Resources

WEBSITES

Center for Mindful Self-Compassion
centerformsc.org

Global Professional Breathwork
Alliance
breathworkalliance.com

Hakomi Institute
hakomiinstitute.com

International Breath Foundation
ibfbreathwork.org

Self-Compassion, Dr. Kristin Neff
self-compassion.org

BOOKS

Accessing the Healing Power of the Vagus Nerve: Self-Help Exercises for Anxiety, Depression, Trauma, and Autism by Stanley Rosenberg

Body-Centered Psychotherapy: The Hakomi Method by Ron Kurtz

The Body Keeps the Score: Brain, Mind, and Body in the Healing of Trauma by Bessel Van Der Kolk

Breath: The New Science of a Lost Art by James Nestor

Breathe Deep, Laugh Loudly: The Joy of Transformational Breathing by Judith Kravitz

Breathe! You Are Alive: Sutra on the Full Awareness of Breathing by Thich Nhat Hanh

Breathing: Expanding Your Power and Energy by Michael Sky

The Breathing Book: Good Health and Vitality Through Essential Breath Work by Donna Farhi

The Healing Power of the Breath: Simple Techniques to Reduce Stress and Anxiety, Enhance Concentration, and Balance Your Emotions by Richard Brown and Patricia Gerbarg

The Mindful Path to Self-Compassion: Freeing Yourself from Destructive Thoughts and Emotions by Christopher Germer

The New Rules of Aging Well: A Simple Program for Immune Resilience, Strength, and Vitality by Frank Lipman, MD, and Danielle Claro

The Oxygen Advantage: Simple, Scientifically Proven Breathing Techniques to Help You Become Healthier, Slimmer, Faster, and Fitter by Patrick McKeown

The Perceptible Breath: A Breathing Science by Ilse Middendorf

Self-Compassion: The Proven Power of Being Kind to Yourself by Kristin Neff

Shaking Medicine: The Healing Power of Ecstatic Movement by Bradford Keeney

The Tao of Natural Breathing: For Health, Well-Being, and Inner Growth by Dennis Lewis

The Way of Rest: Finding the Courage to Hold Everything in Love by Jeff Foster

Acknowledgments

A heartfelt thank-you to my publisher, Lia Ronnen; my editor, Shoshana Gutmajer, who went the extra mile to get this done with great care and unwavering support; and Ellen Morrissey, who jumped in with curiosity and a much-needed clear eye, for all their hard work, skillful shaping, and patience throughout this project. I feel blessed to have worked with such gifted and kind women.

A big thanks to the amazing team at Artisan Books, who carried this book from words to its beautiful form and out into the world: production editor Sibylle Kazeroid, production director Nancy Murray, production assistant Erica Huang, editorial assistant Diana Valcarcel, designer Maggie Byrd, art director Suet Chong, and Katie Acheson Wolford for her beautiful illustrations.

My deepest thanks to Danielle Claro, whose creative spark is contagious and without whom this book would not exist, for her endless support and belief in me and the power of breathwork along with her masterful guidance, editing skill, and lasting friendship. Thank you for your major role in building the structure so that every part of this book could have a home.

Sincere gratitude to my siblings: Therese for being my daily angel, Gay for all the helpful guidance, and Tim and Martha for the encouraging check-ins; your supportive calls, love, and humor were the wind beneath my wings, especially in the moments when I thought I reached my limits, again and again . . . and again.

To my women's group of thirteen years, Deah Baird, Anne Marie Benjamin, Aletha Eastwood, Nova Knutson, and Nina Yates, for being my circle of support and for their input as colleagues and providing sanity through laughter and listening, a deep thank you. Thank you to my dear friends who were there when I needed connection and a consult: Kathy Marchant, Allison Howard, Laurie Cox, Ryan Crosby, Eric Franklin, Sherri Holman, Shari Cordon, Sabena Butler, Roxanne Thomas, and Gary Lawson.

Many thanks to my wellness team, Padeen Quinn, Valerie Vogel, Sharon Woodward, and William Wise, who kept my body and mind going during this project.

A heartfelt thank-you to all my teachers, including Judith Kravitz, Jim Morningstar, John Eisman, Donna Roy, Kristin Neff, and Christopher Germer, whose knowledge and wisdom is infused into my work with every client and into every class I teach. I'm grateful to all the breathwork pioneers and practitioners who came before me and paved the way for me to have a life of practicing and teaching the gift of breath.

Thank you to all my clients through the years who helped me connect to the heart and soul of breathwork and who continue to inspire me to walk my talk.

Index

Library of Congress Cataloging-in-Publication Data

Names: Townsend, Margaret (Breathing facilitator), author.
Title: The breathwork companion : unlock the healing power of breathing / Margaret Townsend.
Description: New York, NY : Artisan, [2023] | Includes index. | Summary: "A practical, accessible guide to our body's greatest wellness resource—the breath"—Provided by publisher.
Identifiers: LCCN 2022033484 | ISBN 9781648290787 (paperback)
Subjects: LCSH: Breathing exercises—Therapeutic use. | Breathing exercises.
Classification: LCC RM733 .T69 2023 | DDC 613/.192—dc23/eng/20220812
LC record available at https://lccn.loc.gov/2022033484

Design by Maggie Byrd

Artisan books are available at special discounts when purchased in bulk for premiums and sales promotions as well as for fundraising or educational use. Special editions or book excerpts also can be created to specification. For details, please contact specialmarkets@hbgusa.com.

Published by Artisan,
an imprint of Workman Publishing Co., Inc.,
a subsidiary of Hachette Book Group, Inc.
1290 Avenue of the Americas, New York, NY 10104
artisanbooks.com

Artisan is a registered trademark of Workman Publishing Co., Inc.,
a subsidiary of Hachette Book Group, Inc.

Printed in China on responsibly sourced paper

First printing, December 2023

1 3 5 7 9 10 8 6 4 2